# The Challenges of Urban Ecological Sanitation

## Praise for this book

'Project failures can contribute to learning as much as any success stories. The sanitation sector has many failures but these are largely unreported. This book is a courageous effort to help us learn from the Erdos project; what can go wrong, so that we can be wiser for our next project. Thanks for the learning opportunity.'
*Jack Sim, Founder, World Toilet Organization*

'Radical sector innovation often encounters great challenges. This book provides a rich and fine-grained account of why and how the acceptance of dry toilet technology in a newly planned neighbourhood in Erdos Eco-Town, China, failed to materialize. It thus contributes important learning for future initiatives in providing more sustainable 'closed-loop' solutions for urban areas.'
*Chris Luethi, Eawag-Sandec, Swiss Federal Institute of Aquatic Science and Technology*

'*The Challenges of Urban Ecological Sanitation* is an excellent account of the best of intentions, diligently pursued, but still flawed in practice. The book sets out a way forward, and lessons learnt, that are an important addition to the efforts to find sanitation solutions which 'close the loop', return nutrients to the soil, save water in scarce areas, and prevent faecal contamination in flood-prone areas. The book is a must-read for those concerned with social engineering, and lesser known technologies in the developing world.'
*Shantha Sheela Nair, Vice Chairman, State Planning Commission, Tamil Nadu, India*

# The Challenges of Urban Ecological Sanitation

## Lessons from the Erdos Eco-Town Project

Arno Rosemarin,
Jennifer McConville,
Amparo Flores, and
Zhu Qiang

PRACTICAL ACTION
Publishing

Practical Action Publishing Ltd
The Schumacher Centre
Bourton on Dunsmore, Rugby,
Warwickshire CV23 9QZ, UK
www.practicalactionpublishing.org



ISBN 9781853397677 Hardback
ISBN 9781853397684 Paperback
ISBN 9781780447674 Library Ebook
ISBN 9781780447681 Ebook



A catalogue record for this book is available from the British Library.



Since 1974, Practical Action Publishing (formerly Intermediate Technology Publications and ITDG Publishing) has published and disseminated books and information in support of international development work throughout the world. Practical Action Publishing is a trading name of Practical Action Publishing Ltd (Company Reg. No. 1159018), the wholly owned publishing company of Practical Action. Practical Action Publishing trades only in support of its parent charity objectives and any profits are covenanted back to Practical Action (Charity Reg. No. 247257, Group VAT Registration No. 880 9924 76).

Cover photo: One of the four-storey buildings in the Erdos Eco-town in Dongsheng City. Photo taken November 2008 by Arno Rosemarin.
Typeset by SJI Services
Printed by Lightning Source

# Contents


| | |
|---|---|
| Figures and boxes | vii |
| Acronyms and abbreviations | ix |
| About the authors | xi |
| Preface | xiii |
| 1. Introduction | 1 |
| Global urban sanitation challenges | 1 |
| Ecological and sustainable sanitation | 4 |
| Motivation for an ecological design in China | 6 |
| Site selection | 7 |
| Project organization | 10 |
| The planning process | 13 |
| Implementation process | 14 |
| 2. Designed to close the loop | 19 |
| Faeces system | 19 |
| Urine system | 27 |
| Greywater system | 30 |
| Solid waste system | 33 |
| 3. Operations and maintenance | 35 |
| Organization | 35 |
| Household level | 36 |
| Systems level | 43 |
| Operating costs | 49 |
| Environmental impacts | 51 |
| Health risks | 52 |
| 4. Research and development | 55 |
| Toilet model improvements | 56 |
| Ventilation retrofitting | 59 |
| Reuse | 61 |
| 5. Social acceptance | 65 |
| Living with dry toilets | 65 |
| Road to flush toilets with onsite treatment | 70 |
| 6. Lessons learned | 73 |
| Institutional arrangements | 74 |
| Technology development | 75 |

Social issues and stakeholders 75
External factors 76
Tipping points 76
Killing factors 77
Lessons learned and ways forward 78

Annex 1. Job descriptions of the project experts 83

Annex 2. Cost-benefit analysis of the EETP ecological sanitation system 85

Acknowledgements 93
Notes 96
References 97

# Figures and boxes

## Figures


| | | |
|---|---|---|
| 1 | Global urban and rural population trends in developing and developed countries | 4 |
| 2 | Location of the Erdos Eco-Town Project in Inner Mongolia in northern China | 8 |
| 3 | Organizational chart of actors involved in planning and executing the EETP | 12 |
| 4 | System diagram of EETP showing the flows for the faeces, urine, and greywater sub-systems | 20 |
| 5 | Structure of the porcelain urine-diverting dry toilet | 21 |
| 6 | The turning mechanism and the bowl | 22 |
| 7 | Illustration of the faeces and urine system | 23 |
| 8 | Two models of the initial lifting mechanism for the bin covers | 24 |
| 9 | Ventilation system showing the toilet, drop chute, collector bin, fan, vent-pipe, and vent-pipe cap | 25 |
| 10 | Cross-section and photograph of the urine-odour trap placed in the porcelain toilet designed to include a thin layer of paraffin oil to help seal the urine from the atmosphere | 28 |
| 11 | Flow chart of the greywater treatment system | 32 |
| 12 | The post-treatment holding pond for greywater | 34 |
| 13 | Management structure for the Erdos Eco-Town Project | 35 |
| 14 | Graphics from the instruction poster on use of the urine-diverting dry toilet and urinal, distributed and explained to each household | 38 |
| 15 | Most common problems reported to the maintenance hotline | 41 |
| 16 | Removal of bins by using a simple hoist installed on a light truck | 44 |
| 17 | Composting plant showing the steps in the process, including material preparation, blending of the effective microorganisms, and actual fermentation | 46 |
| 18 | Cross-sections of the third toilet model, showing the sliding plate design | 57 |
| 19 | The Separett model, with bottom removed, connected to the drop chute, and the removable bottomless pail to ease cleaning | 58 |

20 Third type of vent-pipe arrangement with sealed cabinets housing the faecal bins 60
21 Survey results of user acceptability of applying untreated urine or treated faeces on various types of crops 63
22 Advertising leaflet to market the apartments in the Erdos Eco-Town 66
23 Results from the Spring 2009 survey regarding user perceptions of the dry sanitation system 68
24 Timeline of significant factors during the project 74
A.1 EETP ecosan and conventional sanitation systems 88

## Boxes

1.1 The Gebers Urban Ecosan Project in Stockholm, Sweden 5
3.1 Workers' voices 45
5.1 Residents' voices 69

# Acronyms and abbreviations

| | |
|---|---|
| CBA | Cost-benefit analysis |
| COD | Chemical oxidation demand |
| DPO | Dongsheng Project Office |
| DS | Dongsheng |
| DEWATS | Decentralized wastewater treatment system |
| Ecosan | Ecological sanitation |
| EcoSanRes | Ecological Sanitation Research |
| EETP | Erdos Eco-Town Project |
| ENPV | Economic net present value |
| GIZ | German Agency for International Cooperation (formerly GTZ, German Agency for Technical Cooperation) |
| GDP | Gross domestic product |
| GWP | Global warming potential |
| HZK | Haozhaokui (location for the EETP) |
| O&M | Operations and maintenance |
| PVC | Polyvinylchloride |
| R&D | Research and development |
| RMB | Renminbi (Yuan Chinese monetary currency) |
| SEI | Stockholm Environment Institute |
| SPO | SEI Project Office |
| STP | Sewage treatment plant |
| SuSanA | Sustainable Sanitation Alliance |
| TAES | Tianjin Academy of Environmental Science |
| TEP | Terrestrial ecotoxicity potential |
| UD | Urine-diverting |
| UDDT | Urine-diverting dry toilet |
| UNDP | United Nations Development Programme |
| UNESCO | United Nations Educational, Scientific, and Cultural Organization |
| UNFPA | United Nations Population Fund |
| UNICEF | United Nations International Children's Emergency Fund |
| USTB | University of Science and Technology Beijing |
| WHO | World Health Organization |
| WWTP | Wastewater treatment plant |

# About the authors

**Arno Rosemarin** (PhD) is Senior Research Fellow at Stockholm Environment Institute (SEI), an aquatic biologist with experience in eutrophication of freshwater and coastal waters, and an expert in ecological sanitation. He was the SEI Project Supervisor of the Erdos Eco-Town Project.

**Jennifer McConville** (PhD) was Researcher at SEI while writing this book. She is a civil engineer and specialist in planning of sustainable sanitation systems, and is currently at CIT Urban Water Management AB, Sweden.

**Amparo Flores** (PhD) did her doctoral thesis at Cambridge University, UK, using the Erdos project as a case study. She is an Associate Engineer at Zone 7 Water Agency in Livermore, California.

**Zhu Qiang** is Professor at Gansu Research Institute for Water Conservancy, China, and an expert in rainwater harvesting, sustainable water and sanitation systems. He was the SEI Senior Advisor to the Erdos Eco-Town Project.

# Preface

The China–Sweden Erdos Eco-Town Project was initiated in 2003 by the Dongsheng District Government and SEI as part of the Ecological Sanitation Research (EcoSanRes) Programme (Dongsheng District Government, 2007). It has involved a large number of collaborating organizations, specialists, and support staff from China, Sweden, Germany, the UK, and Japan to introduce and develop source-separation sanitation techniques in modern four- and five-storey apartment buildings in this semi-arid zone of northern China. The objective was to carry out a research and development (R&D) project but also to do this at full scale in order to deal with the reality of full implementation with 3,000 inhabitants. The first phase of the project, the subject of this book, was completed in 2006 and consisted of building 832 apartments in 42 buildings as a new housing project in the quickly growing city of Dongsheng in Erdos Municipality in Inner Mongolia, China.

Dongsheng District is located within the Yellow River drainage basin in the south-western part of Inner Mongolia and the central part of the Erdos plateau at an altitude of 1,400–1,600 m above sea level. The city is located in a major coal-mining and natural gas region with a temperate, semi-arid climate, an annual precipitation of *ca* 50–400 mm, about 2,000 mm in potential evapo-transpiration, air temperatures ranging from –30 to +30°C, and ground freezing to 1.5 m depth.

The population of Dongsheng is presently about 500,000 and is part of Erdos municipality (1.5 million inhabitants), one of the fastest growing urban areas in China (Woodworth, 2011; World Bank, 2005). At the start of the project in 2003, the population was only about 250,000 and the downtown area consisted of about 60,000 households, 15,000 in multi-storey and 45,000 in single-storey buildings, of which one-third had private flush toilets and two-thirds used public toilets, mainly dingy pit latrines. In the peri-urban and surrounding semi-rural areas, most households had and continue to have private, shallow-pit latrines – most of which are in miserable condition, and open defecation still exists.

In 2003, at the start of the project, about one-third of the city was forced to ration water with three to four hours of interspersed supply per day. The main source of water supply is from groundwater at *ca* 30 m depth. Prior to 1985, when collector pipes were introduced to the city centre, household sewage, including flush toilet waste, was jointly discharged with storm water through open trenches. The practices observed in 2003 at the start of the project contributed to polluting the groundwater and there was an obvious need for a more sustainable system to help prevent pollution and conserve water. It is against this background that the city decided to test and develop ecological sanitation (ecosan) dry toilets in multi-storey buildings.

Urban dry sanitation has been tried in a few demonstration projects, for example in China, South Africa, Sweden, and Germany (Berger and Lorenz-Ladener, 2008). The Erdos project represents the first attempt at a full-scale project. The eco-town was equipped with modern porcelain toilets and urinals using design standards developed in Sweden and China. The sanitation approach used in this project involved urine-diverting dry toilets (UDDTs) connected by a chute (280 mm diameter) to basement collection wheelie bins (120 l) for faeces and sawdust (compostable sorbent) placed in ventilated, sealed cabinets. Although based on proven technology from the 'Gebers' project in Sweden (Palmqvist and Jönsson, 2003) the application to four to five storeys was new.

The stakes were high at the onset of the project, knowing that there were no building design standards nor was there access to skilled labour with experience in dry sanitation systems. The project adapted as well as possible to the local conditions. This book tells the story of the Erdos Eco-Town Project: a Chinese experiment in urban ecological sanitation.

This book is written for a wide audience. In particular it is relevant for practitioners, researchers, and policy-makers working in the area of water, sanitation, and hygiene in both developed and developing countries. Specialists working on ecosan, UDDTs, and innovative sanitation solutions will be especially interested in this book. It is also of interest to sanitation engineers working in particular with urban solutions.

# CHAPTER 1
# Introduction

The Erdos[1] Eco-Town Project (EETP) came into being as a result of a number of global and national needs and pressures to improve methods for handling human waste streams in urban areas. The initiative for a major urban sanitation project in China using alternative approaches came from the Swedish International Development Cooperation Agency (SIDA) within the EcoSanRes Programme (www.ecosanres.org) managed by SEI. This sanitation programme, which ran from 2001 to 2011, was designed to promote pro-poor sanitation solutions by developing and disseminating evidence-based research. The programme aimed to contribute to efforts to improve the global sanitation situation in ways that were both environment friendly and sustainable. As one of the fastest-growing transition economies and the world's most populous country, China is a key target for building collaboration and carrying out ambitious pilot projects. The extreme water shortages in northern China beckon the development of alternative and more sustainable sanitation systems that save on water use and allow for reuse of the various products.

Much progress has been made over recent years in the area of ecosan. A global survey carried out by the German Agency for Technical Cooperation (GTZ – which is now the German Agency for International Cooperation, GIZ) and updated to 2011 showed that there have been 315 recorded ecosan projects involving 4.8 million people in some 70 countries. The majority of these have been rural and peri-urban projects. Urban demonstration projects have been ongoing for the past 10–15 years in several countries: Sweden, Germany, Switzerland, Mexico, Philippines, Bolivia, Ethiopia, Uganda, Burkina Faso, Kenya, South Africa, India, Nepal, China, and elsewhere. Case histories have been documented and published by the Sustainable Sanitation Alliance (SuSanA). Policy breakthroughs have been achieved whereby sustainable sanitation has been included in the overall sanitation development policy in South-east Asia with the Manila Declaration signed in 2010 by the participating ministers from 13 countries. Also in India in 2010 the Total Sanitation Campaign (TSC) Guidelines were amended to include ecosan. Indeed, in China, which has most of the world's ecosan installations, dry sanitation with urine diversion has become a standard option in rural and peri-urban areas.

## Global urban sanitation challenges

Half of the world population is now urban and most of the future population growth in the world will be in urban settings (United Nations Population Fund [UNFPA], 2007; Rosemarin, 2005). Conventional sewerage approaches to urban sanitation have had major success in the developed world, especially when it comes to improved hygiene safety for the users, but these systems have proven to be more difficult to maintain in the developing countries (Black and Fawcett, 2008; Rosemarin, 2007). Challenges surrounding urban sanitation are particularly aggravated in arid parts of the world with water-supply shortages but even in areas with high precipitation and poor drainage where sewer pipes and pit latrines become inundated with drainage water for lengthy periods. Innovation in urban centres involves rethinking the omnipresent centralized systems that use large-bore sewer pipes and often combined drainage/runoff and sewage systems. Few projects have attempted to use dry urine-diverting systems in urban dwellings and the technology is relatively new especially in multi-storey buildings. The economics of semi-manual collection of human excreta may be similar to those of urban solid waste although this has not been fully investigated. Landfills and garbage dumps for mixed solid waste are an enormous burden for municipalities and therefore more advanced systems involving source separation, composting, and incineration are being adopted in order to reduce the mammoth volumes (Williams, 2005). At population densities from 150–200 inhabitants per hectare, waterborne sewage in piped systems starts to become more economic than individual on site systems that require manual or semi-manual emptying (Mara, 1998). This is especially true if the sewerage system is designed using small-bore pipes and with simplified treatment systems, such as a decentralized wastewater treatment system (DEWATS) (BORDA, 2009).

As fertilizer prices continue to increase, the potential value of sanitation nutrient sources to urban agriculture increases, especially for the poorest parts of countries and where transportation costs make fertilizers even more expensive (Rosemarin *et al.* 2008). Phosphorus resources are limited and getting more expensive (Rosemarin *et al.* 2009) and this will soon force many countries around the world to revalue the urban streams of organic material from kitchen and sanitation sources and to introduce reuse systems. Dry and low-water systems will have, in many cases, major advantages over the ones designed around large water volumes.

Providing sanitation services to the world's poor remains one of the greatest challenges in international development. For the 2.6 billion people without access to improved sanitation services, this lack increases their risk of disease, reduces their quality of life and negatively affects their opportunities for economic advancement (WHO & UNICEF, 2008). The effects from poor sanitation are not only a problem for the poor, but have wider impacts as the release of extra nutrients cause eutrophication and fish kills in aquatic environments.

Recognition of the urgency of the global sanitation situation is growing. In 2002, sanitation targets were added to the list of Millennium Development Goals (MDG), originally set by the UN in 2000. The United Nations Development Programme (UNDP) featured water and sanitation in the Human Development report of 2006 and the UN declared 2008 as the

International Year of Sanitation (IYS). However, the challenge of meeting the MDG target for improved sanitation, let alone sanitation that prevents environmental contamination, remains huge. There are 2.6 billion people in the world without access to proper sanitation, making the sanitation target the largest of all MDGs in terms of population; double that of targets like water supply and malnutrition, and dwarfing any of the health targets like malaria, HIV/AIDS, and TB (Rosemarin *et al.*, 2008). Yet, these numbers are based on a definition of improved sanitation that does not strictly take into account the downstream environmental and health consequences of dysfunctional or incomplete treatment schemes. The real impacts of poor sanitation may be even larger. Over 700 million people in 50 countries are consuming foodstuffs that have been irrigated with untreated sewage (Scott *et al.*, 2004), and half of the world population is infected with parasites linked to poor sanitation conditions affecting food, water, and the living environment (Chan, 1997; Capron *et al.*, 2004; Miguel and Kremer, 2004; United Nations Educational, Scientific and Cultural Organization [UNESCO], 2006). Moreover, the situation is being exacerbated by the increasing urbanization trends that concentrate people and their waste products in increasingly dense areas (SuSanA, 2008).

The need for improved sanitation is most critical and will perhaps have the greatest impact in densely populated urban and peri-urban areas. Health risks from poor sanitation are greatest in urban areas where high population density in contaminated areas facilitates the transfer of disease. The global population is becoming more and more urban (Figure 1), especially in developing countries where sanitation solutions are generally missing or insufficient. The result is a conglomeration of wastewater, most of which is released without adequate treatment (Ujang and Henze, 2006). In addition, slum populations, many without access to either water or sanitation services, continue to increase, now running at more than one-third of the urban population (UN Habitat, 2008). The urban sanitation challenge is thus to find a way to meet the needs of a vast population in a dignified manner that does not add to the global environmental burden.

This challenge will require sanitation solutions that are resource-efficient and interlinked with other urban services. Conventional modern wastewater treatment plants, if built and maintained properly, can be effective systems for protecting human health and providing a cleaner environment, thereby achieving the main objective of a sanitation system. As the world becomes more aware of the interlinkages and complexities involved in protecting the natural environment, e.g. the issues of climate change, over consumption, and dwindling natural resources, the conventional systems are being criticized as unsustainable (Lüthi *et al.*, 2010). The indiscriminate release of fertilizing nutrients such as nitrogen and phosphorus from wastewater flows is an increasing concern that links strongly to agricultural demand for limited global phosphorus reserves (Rosemarin *et al.*, 2009; Rosemarin *et al.*, 2010). There is an increasing demand for innovations that will conserve water, use energy more efficiently, and reuse the nutrients found in the waste streams.

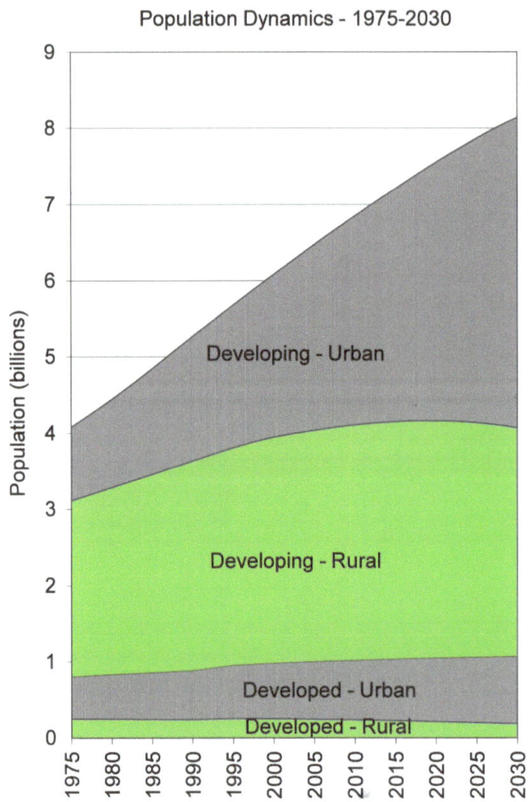


**Figure 1.** Global urban and rural population trends in developing and developed countries
*Source:* based on World Population Prospects: The 2006 Revision, medium variant

## Ecological and sustainable sanitation

Ecological sanitation has been developed in response to strong global drivers for improving the way that waste is handled in society. The concept of ecosan is based on closing the loop on nutrient and water cycles by recycling the residual products (excreta, solid waste, and water). Ecosan systems safely recycle excreta and other organic waste products back to crop production in such a way that the use of non-renewable resources is minimized. The objective is to protect human health and the environment while reducing the use of water in sanitation systems and recycling nutrients to help reduce the need for chemical fertilizers in agriculture. Ecosan represents a conceptual shift in the relationship between people and the environment; it is built on the necessary link between people and soil.

A key concept for working with ecological sanitation is an understanding that the sanitation system is more than technical infrastructure, and that a functional system is also reliant on individuals and management frameworks that control the operation and maintenance along the entire treatment process. A sanitation system thus encompasses the institutions regulating the system, the organization and management, the users, and the entire technical infrastructure required to achieve collection, transport, treatment, and management of end products of human excreta, greywater, solid waste, stormwater drainage, and industrial and agricultural waste products. A sustainable sanitation system is one that protects and promotes human health, minimizes environmental degradation and depletion of the resource base, and is technically and institutionally appropriate, socially acceptable, and economically viable also in the long term (SuSanA, 2008). Ecological sanitation focuses on the health, environment, and resource aspects of sustainable sanitation. Ecological sanitation systems can be implemented in a sustainable way if technical, institutional, social, and economical aspects are cared for appropriately.

At the start of the Erdos Eco-Town Project in 2003, the concept of ecological sanitation had been successfully applied in several villages in China, notably in Guangxi Province (EcoSanRes, 2004). There were, however, few urban applications of the concept. The project's hypothesis was that the ecosan concept could be applied in a cost-effective way by bringing residual products from households and workplaces to 'eco-stations' serving the community. In this way the project was to demonstrate sustainable approaches to sanitation, water use, solid waste management and infrastructure within an urban community (EcoSanRes, 2004). It set out to establish an ecological and sustainable four-step process for dealing with human excreta: (1) source-separation; (2) containment; (3) sanitization; and (4) recycling. Source-separation of waste flows (faeces, urine, wash water and solid waste) facilitates application of the ecosan concept. For example, since the majority of harmful bacteria and viruses in human excreta are found in faeces, separation of urine can significantly reduce the volume of waste that needs active or long-term treatment, as well as facilitate the recycling of nutrients through use of urine as a liquid

**Box 1.1 The Gebers Urban Ecosan Project in Stockholm, Sweden**

The Erdos project was inspired by the well-functioning urine-diverting dry toilet project in Stockholm located at the Gebers housing complex. Here, 32 families have been using dry toilets installed in this two-storey building since 1997. Urine is piped to storage tanks that are emptied with a suction truck and driven to a local farmer. The faeces are collected in ventilated bins in the basement after a straight drop from the toilet. These are sanitized through storage-composting. Organic household waste is also composted.

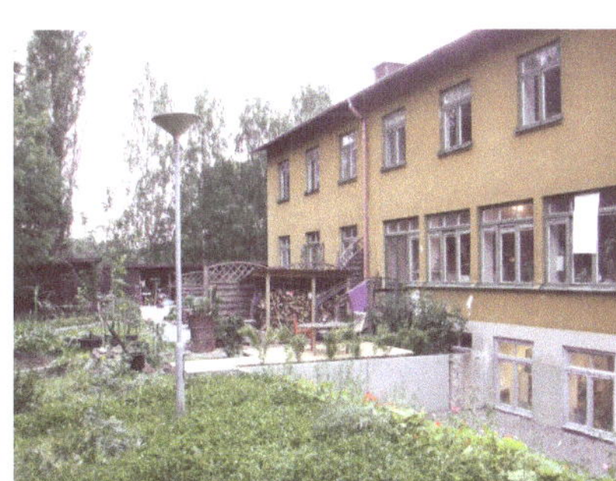

Photo: Ian Caldwell, SEI

fertilizer. Once the waste flows are separated they can be contained and treated to acceptable levels for reuse. Development of a suitable ecosan system for urban areas was the main driver for the Erdos Eco-Town Project.

## Motivation for an ecological design in China

China is rapidly urbanizing and putting increasing strain on urban infrastructure and services, particularly sanitation. According to 2008 statistics, the Chinese population was 43 per cent urban and only 58 per cent of urban residents had access to improved sanitation (WHO and UNICEF, 2010). Of the wastewater collected from those urban residents only 50 per cent was treated (World Bank, 2007). This increased to 59 per cent in 2008, according to official statistics (Innovation Centre Denmark–Shanghai, 2009) and it should be remembered that this is essentially primary treatment with limited or no removal of phosphate or nitrate. The neglect of the sanitation sector perhaps mirrors what has been the rather negative global environmental reputation that China gained during its economic rise in the last few decades. The EETP was conceived at a time when China had already undergone more than two decades of rapid economic development. China is presently at a crossroads where choices have to be made on how to sustain continued economic development while not sacrificing the environment, draining the resources base, or exacerbating the already alarming disparities between the rich and poor, and rural and urban areas. As a result, a development paradigm shift was urgently called for by institutionalizing the 'scientific development concept'[2]. This has allowed China to make tremendous efforts to improve its environmental legislation and promote ecological programmes. A number of special eco-cities have been built, setting special emphasis on sustainability. The 'recycling economy' has become the national policy of China, resulting in a major push at various levels of government to make laws and start projects related to saving water resources and recycling.

From an ecological sanitation perspective, China has a long history of using human waste as fertilizer. Prior to the 1960s, Chinese farmers relied almost exclusively on organic fertilizers. With the advent of chemical fertilizers in the 1970s, the use of organic fertilizer decreased, but environmental awareness and a growing demand for organic produce means that the demand for organic fertilizers is on the rise again. In 2007 there were 2,282 organic fertilizer companies in China treating sludge and organic wastes, including faecal sludge, running at about 50 per cent capacity (Bai, 2009). Farmers are encouraged to apply good-quality organic manure, including treated faeces and urine, supplemented with chemical fertilizers and to use green manure. There are also policies in place that encourage the construction of ecological sanitation systems through investment and preferential policies.

In the beginning of the 2000s, based on the success of the ecosan pilot projects in Guangxi Province carried out by Lin Jiang and Uno Winblad and the promising policy situation, EcoSanRes decided to continue the ecological sanitation promotion in China by establishing a large urban pilot project. The rationale for such a decision was straightforward and could not have been any stronger, even to this day. Globally, alternative and sustainable urban sanitation systems and solutions are desperately needed and development and testing is necessary. Despite small-scale successful examples, no proven large-scale implementation yet exists. Among many other reasons, one major obstacle for large-scale urban application is the fact that, at least in the industrialized countries, it is very difficult and costly to deviate from the existing waterborne sewage systems. Conversely, the rapidly urbanizing developing countries offer the 'building-from-scratch' opportunity that many argue is critical for testing the alternative urban sanitation systems. In addition to the positive historical and cultural environment for reuse of human waste in China as mentioned, growing water scarcity, rapid urbanization, and the policy push for building the 'resource-saving and environment-friendly society' are some of the other factors that justified the choice of establishing this urban sanitation pilot project.

To select a suitable location required additional criteria, however. Firstly, it had to be in the 'emerging cities' category, where no existing sewage system was already installed, and in a zone of severe water shortage. Secondly, it had to have a local government that not only shared the vision and significance of the pilot project but also showed a strong will to support and participate. Third and no less important was the need for a specific local urban development plan that was in the pipeline and compatible with the designed project size as well as the basic elements of R&D and testing.

Those criteria and a two-year search and site investigation process eventually led to the project site in Dongsheng District, Erdos City, Inner Mongolia Autonomous Region and the establishment of the Erdos Eco-Town Project.

## Site selection

At the beginning of 2003, a project-site investigation mission was organized to Erdos City, Inner Mongolia, and to Zhangjiakou City, Hebei Province, both in northern China where water scarcity is a major concern and urbanization is rapid. In Erdos, the team visited three potential sites in Dalad Banner, EjinHoro Banner, and Dongsheng District. In the end, a rural–urban farmer resettlement project at a location called Haozhaokui in Dongsheng District (Figure 2) was deemed by the team as the most interesting and suitable potential project site for the urban ecological sanitation pilot testing and development.

The Haozhaokui project location had already been identified by the Dongsheng District to resettle the farmers who had lost their land to urban expansion. This is an area of about 20–30 km$^2$, located in the north-west part of the 'future city' according to the city master plan for 2020. Yet, at the time, it was still quite a distance from the existing city centre and was mainly hillside farmland occupied by only a few households of the Haozhaokui Village. The original Dongsheng District plan was to have 1,000 households resettled into

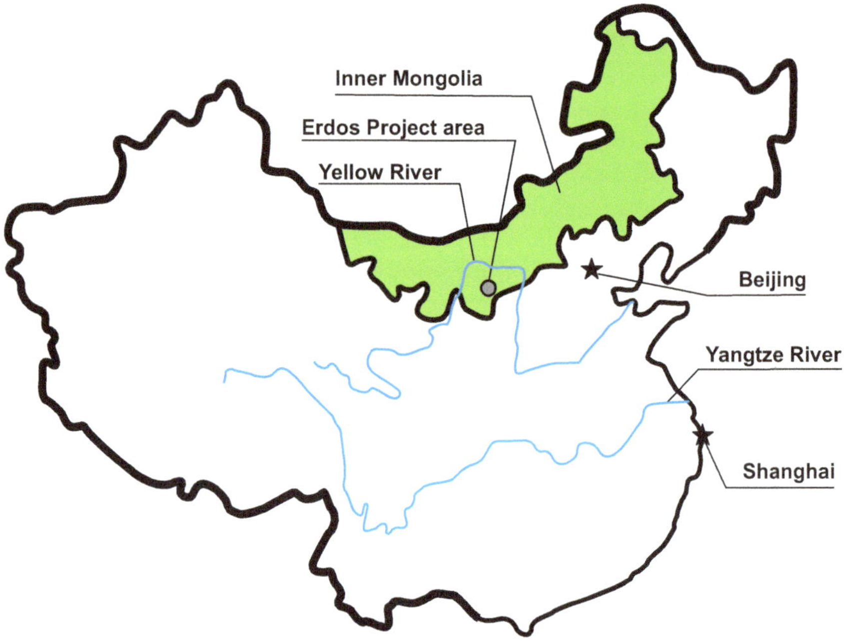


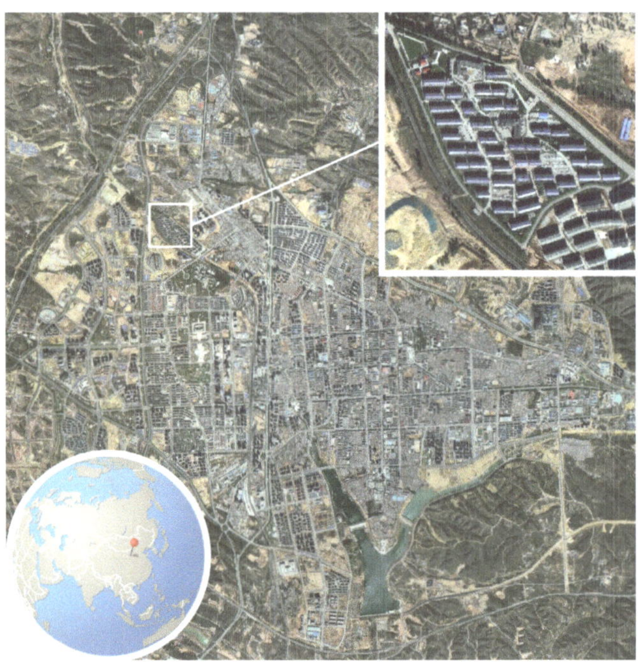

©2012 Google

**Figure 2.** Location of the Erdos Eco-Town Project in Inner Mongolia in northern China (above) and aerial view over Dongsheng City (below). The location of the EETP is the smaller insert
*Source:* Google Earth

the area before the end of 2005. About 230 buildings in the area had been planned and were to be designed in 2003 and the construction was to start from June 2003. The original plan was to build simple one- and two-storey courtyard houses which are common in small urban centres in China.

When the ecosan system concept was presented to the local government, it was received with great enthusiasm, especially since the local government was seeking examples of good environmental performance on the one hand, and suffering from extreme water shortage hindering its rapid urbanization on the other. After three consecutive years of severe drought from 1999 to 2001, combined with rapid urban expansion, Dongsheng City was experiencing its most severe water shortage ever. Urban residential water supply was rationed and available for a fixed number of hours each day. In addition, the strong endorsement of the project by the local government enhanced the vision of providing the world with the first major urban ecosan model that would draw attention not only from China but globally.

### *Background on Dongsheng City*

Dongsheng City is a district of Erdos Municipality in Inner Mongolia, northern China. The location is in the Yellow River drainage basin in northern China, Inner Mongolia, an area characterized by water shortage and cold seasonal climate. Once a municipality itself, Dongsheng is the political, economic, and cultural centre of Erdos Municipality. At the start of the project, the population of the entire Erdos Municipality was about 1.3 million, and that of the Dongsheng District was 250,000. There had been a significant urbanization trend in the city since the 1990s which led to a decline in the population of the surrounding small towns and villages. The District is rich in natural resources and coal mining is one of the most important industries. Coal mining in the area at the rate of 250–300 million tons per year is one of the major drivers behind economic development and the subsequent urbanization in the area. Agriculture production is still considered one of the five economic pillars of the district, however at a significantly lower scale than industrial production. In 2000, total agricultural and total industrial production was valued at 120 million and 6.33 billion Renminbi (RMB), respectively (EcoSanRes, 2004) (7.4 RMB to US$1 as at January 2012). The average disposable income of urban residents at this time was 6,000 RMB while that of rural residents was 2,368 RMB (ibid.). It was envisioned at the start of the project that many of the future residents of the eco-town would be rural farmers who were resettled into cities. The government-organized rural–urban migration or resettlement has been one of the main local strategies integrating poverty reduction, grassland restoration, and promotion of urbanization and industrialization since 2000. For farmers who had been resettled because of urban expansion, like those who were originally the targeted residents of the Haozhaokui project, they could get a compensation of 20,000 RMB for each mu of arable land and 10,000 RMB for each mu of non-arable land (the Chinese measurement unit for area, 15 mu = 1 ha.) The usual land ownership per person was about 10 mu in the area, so there was some incentive to move to the city.

The northern part of China is one of the most water-stressed in the world with annual precipitation ranging from less than 50 mm up to 400 mm per year and annual evapo-transpiration rates of around 2,000 mm ranging between 1,170 and 2,704 mm (Ma *et al.*, 2007). The climate is typical of temperate, continental, semi-arid areas with a characteristically dry and often windy spring, a short warm and often wet summer, a cool autumn, and long and cold winter. Rainfall is highly variable and dry spells can last for months so that all rivers and streams in the area are seasonal.

In such a climate, the rapid urbanization due to industrialization from mineral extraction has put extreme pressure on water resources. The water supply at the start of the project was essentially from groundwater extraction and amounted to 28,000 t/day, which could not meet the demand (EcoSanRes, 2004). Annual water availability ran between 350 and 750 $m^3$ per capita, well below the critical level of 1,000 which defines water scarcity (Shalizi, 2006).

In 2002 the first sewage treatment plant (STP) was put into operation with a daily capacity of 30,000 $m^3$, but due to inadequate collector pipe coverage, the volume treated was about 50 per cent of capacity.

About one-third of the Dongsheng District was forced to ration water: it was made available three times per day for periods of 60–90 minutes. At the start of the project, the main source of drinking water was from fossil groundwater aquifers, supplemented by seasonal surface water sources. Plans were in place, however, for a 100 km pipeline from the Yellow River that would supply 100,000 t/day of water to the city. Even with the new water supply the price of water in Erdos was still predicted to be high, as much as 3–4 RMB (\$0.35–0.50)/$m^3$. About one-third of Erdos households had flush toilets while the rest of the population used the 300 public pit latrines, most of which were without lighting or heating. The poor sanitation conditions taxed further the already impoverished water supply situation by contributing pathogens and nutrients to groundwater pollution. It is against this background that the city decided to test and develop ecosan dry toilets in multi-storey buildings.

While the project was ongoing, development of the city's sewage treatment capacity was initiated. The original STP from 2002 was expanded in 2005 to 40,000 $m^3$/day using a two-stage aerated bio-film process but was still running at less than 75 per cent capacity in 2008. As of 2007, approximately 75 per cent of Dongsheng's urban area was covered by the sewer system. An additional treatment plant of similar capacity (40,000 $m^3$/d) was built in 2009 to meet the city's rapid growth.

## Project organization

The China–Sweden Erdos Eco-Town Project was organized as a collaboration between the Dongsheng District Government and the SEI. A Letter of Intent for the EETP was signed between Erdos Municipality and SEI in March 2003.

Plans changed swiftly, however, in this bustling urban area. The original idea of individual courtyard housing was shifted to standard four- and five-storey apartment buildings. The project was no longer one targeted to displaced farmers but to the open market. The market for urban housing began to expand in Dongsheng much like most other urban centres in China. An added factor was the increased value of coal which provided a new impetus to expansion and modernization. During the course of the project coal prices tripled and the population of Dongsheng increased by over 50 per cent.

The project agreement that was signed 23 September 2003 committed the two parties to the goal of carrying out 'a full-scale implementation project with research and development involving recycling of human excreta, household solid and organic wastes, and greywater [that would] provide China and the world with a sustainable ecological town to learn from and to study'. Within this agreement it was specified that SEI would fund the project preparation, research and development work, training, and demonstration of the different components. The Dongsheng District commitment was to fund the land, labour, building materials, and local administration and management. The building company (Daxing Estate Development Company) signed an agreement with the Dongsheng Government to construct the buildings and install the entire ecosan system according to design. Daxing agreed to finance the construction, with the exception of installation of water supply, electricity, heating, communication, and natural gas which was carried out by the Dongsheng Government. Daxing was given responsibility to sell the houses/apartments at market prices. The Erdos Design Institute provided the approved blueprints in order to follow building norms. SEI examined the blueprints, to ensure that the ecosan installations were designed according to plan, although these were often delivered after the construction had been started.

The project was managed by the Government of Dongsheng with collaborative supervisory and advisory support by SEI. Each side provided personnel in order to carry out the project. SEI added Chinese and external specialists to carry out specific tasks and various R&D studies. The project document was finalized in June 2004 providing the direction and details to be undertaken. The original goal was to hand over the project by the end of 2007 but in actual fact it was finalized in 2009. An international sustainable sanitation conference attended by 500 people was held in Dongsheng in 2007 to showcase the project (www.ecosanres.org/icss/). A workshop was held in 2009 to review the lessons learned from the project (www.ecosanres.org/erdosworkshop2009.htm).

A missing link that lacked transparency was the inspection of the buildings by the Construction Bureau and its designated inspection companies. This turned out to be of considerable importance since the building project was riddled with inadequacies, illegal pipe and electrical connections, buildings without drainage, and pipes without insulation and these were a major cause of faulty function in the plumbing and ventilation systems. The construction and plumbing were sub-contracted to several firms in order to save time and the calibre of the work therefore varied. Building inspection was essentially non-existent and inadequacies in construction were discovered well after the buildings and installations were completed. It was not until the tenants had been living in their flats for about two years that the faulty piping was discovered by opening up walls and ceilings.

The project was run by a Project Manager appointed by the Dongsheng District (Figure 3). This was the Head of the Environment Protection Bureau. SEI provided a Project Supervisor, two Senior Advisors, a Project Manager and assistant staff within the SEI Project Office (SPO). The District provided staff to man the Dongsheng Project Office (DPO), administrative staff, and team members for the various work teams. SEI provided external research experts (both Chinese and foreign) for each work team for training, advisory services and to carry out R&D work.

The management system included the SEI Project team, the DS Government and its representative the DS Project Office, the Building Contractor and the (architectural) Design Institute. Governance was provided by the Steering Committee (SC) composed of senior representatives from the above three main bodies plus the Communist Party Secretary. They met only a few times and did not intervene to solve conflicts or challenges. In effect the governing body was the office of the Mayor of Dongsheng District and the mayors (four altogether during the course of the project) had close contact with the project throughout. Internal information flow was a challenge also complicated by the need to use simultaneous translation between Chinese and English. Also

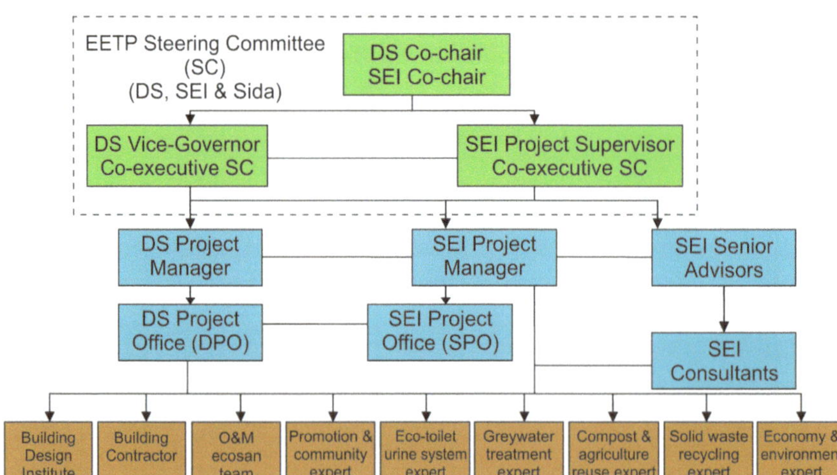


**Figure 3.** Organizational chart of actors involved in planning and executing the Erdos Eco-Town Project (EETP). DS=Dongsheng; SEI=Stockholm Environment Institute

delegation of responsibilities was difficult on the Chinese side since most decisions took on a characteristic top-down nature.

The level of interest taken by the office of the Mayor was highest at the commencement of the project. With each change in mayor, a new learning curve was necessary, and other projects of a larger nature came into play as the city experienced a huge building boom. The shift in standard of living in Erdos during this project was nothing short of phenomenal and exemplary of what uncontrolled development of oil and gas can do to housing markets. Dongsheng went from one of the poorest urban centres to having a gross domestic product (GDP) level higher than Hong Kong's within five years (Want China Times, 2011). This fast growth spurred the local government to raise the stakes and build a new neighbouring city, Kangbashi, with housing and infrastructure for a million inhabitants. The idea of learning how to save water through an experimental dry toilet project for 3,000 people in Dongsheng was now thoroughly dwarfed by the super-ambitious plans to build more and more. The harsh realities of the market place presented themselves, however, with Kangbashi, presently a ghost town, only attracting some 20,000 people. Finally in 2011 the region experienced a collapse in the housing market.

## The planning process

The project was planned in an open manner involving the staff from the municipal government, Design Institute and eventually the building company (Daxing Estate Development Co.) once they were brought into the project. Teams were organized in order to divide the various components into specialist groups.

At an early stage, even prior to signing the project agreements, visits were made to Sweden to examine several urban ecosan projects. These included ones with low-consumption and no-mix waterborne as well as dry urine-diverting systems. The decision to go ahead with the dry system was taken by the then Mayor Zhang Dongsheng in 2003. This would maximize the water savings capacity of the system to be developed. Mayor Zhang was in many ways the visionary and father to this project. He was inspired by what he saw in Sweden, particularly when visiting the successful UDDT apartment complex (Gebers – see Box 1.1) in southern Stockholm. The Gebers two-storey apartment complex at that point had existed for more than seven years and was a clear success.

The toilet used in the Erdos project received a lot of attention from the start and it was designed and tested at an early stage before planning and implementation. Development and testing of an appropriate toilet for the multi-storey installations was initiated in Sweden and prototypes were then transferred to a number of households in the Dongsheng area for further testing and improvements. Ventilation was based on the Gebers design but modified for four- and five-storey buildings. Chinese ventilation experts were brought in to design this system. Originally four buildings were designated for testing prior to implementation, but the building company decided to speed up this procedure since the market pressure was so strong. Without this important period of testing and development, the faeces collection bins and ventilation piping arrangement were installed in all the buildings only to be upgraded and retrofitted a few years later.

Greywater treatment was an issue that required added attention since the Swedish experts offered a design based on oxygenated biofilm treatment on fixed substrate that was not found acceptable by the Chinese authorities. Prior to the implementation of the EETP project, a workshop of Swedish and Chinese experts was held to discuss options for greywater management in cold regions. Originally, the Norwegian 'Spray-filtration' technique was suggested as the greywater treatment solution for EETP by the Swedish consultant. Greywater from the households was to be collected by the piping system to be taken to the eco-station and then treated. However, an evaluation by the Chinese partners found that although the O&M of this technique is simpler, the initial cost for the fixed substrate ('leca' furnaced clay aggregates) was very high compared to the conventional wastewater treatment technique adopted commonly in China plus the large building area was prohibitive. The project therefore opted for a standard treatment plant designed by the Tianjin Academy of Environmental Sciences.

Detailed job descriptions were agreed upon for the various project experts as listed in Annex 1.

A number of R&D projects were carried out within the project, as follows:

- cost-benefit analysis (CBA) comparing the ecological sanitation system with a conventional one of similar capacity (summary paper included as Annex 2 to this book);
- ventilation system assessment and recommendations;
- greywater treatment and collection system;
- composting system;
- agriculture reuse of the products from the ecological sanitation system;
- environmental impact assessment using life-cycle analysis;
- toilet design improvements;
- sterilization of sawdust;
- cleaning methods to remove struvite in urine pipes and odour traps.

## Implementation process

This ecosan project was a unique private–public partnership in which the private developer (Daxing Estate Development Company) adapted a sustainable sanitation approach in a real-estate business venture in return for access to the land area for the project and a promised government tax rebate. The result provided a per $m^2$ cost of about 1,000 RMB in 2006 when the apartments were sold, which was about 30 per cent less than the going rate in the central downtown area for new housing. The apartments were all sold in a short period of time on the open market. Each household signed an agreement accepting the responsibility of using a dry toilet.

Demonstration, training, and state-of-the-art ecosan knowledge was provided by the EcoSanRes Programme at SEI. The R&D ecosan support related to technical solutions, management aspects, institutional dimensions, community sensitization, policy promotion, large-scale agro-reuse demonstrations, cost-benefit analyses, and monitoring. Training of the various stakeholders was provided by SEI at the onset as well as throughout the first years of the project. This involved hands-on demonstration for the government, building company, maintenance team, and households.

The project was characterized by several weaknesses in part relating to the lack of capacity of the building company but also the lack of official building inspection. In general there was a lack of skilled labour especially when it came to plumbing and electrical work. Deviations occurred in the implementation of the building blueprints, for example in the placement of urine and ventilation pipes, causing sub-standard fittings and leakages, a major source of odour. Once an inventory of the many building errors was carried out and a model retrofitting carried out, the building company was unwilling to take on this added responsibility and expense.

The project was in a way a 'living laboratory' for the *ca* 3,000 inhabitants. A hotline was set up in order to provide same-day service but also to collect data on what hardware was malfunctioning or if odour was a problem. The project underwent a number of retrofits to improve toilet ventilation and urine-odour management as the knowledge base grew. A number of households (about 20) had initially 'illegally' installed flush toilets and connected them to the urine pipe system. These were never removed by the government and contributed to the increasing opinion that flush toilets were an alternative worth striving for after a few years of habitation. When interviewed, households acknowledged that the dry system could save valuable water, and reduce pollution load but they also retained the attitude that dry toilets were something for rural communities and not for modern urban multi-storey apartments. The weakest link in this project has been the lack of strong ownership on behalf of the households which eventually expressed itself in terms of user resistance. A general comment has been that the toilets have been awkward to use and that explaining their function to visiting relatives and friends was considered an embarrassment and unnecessary burden. Other complaints centred around the use of sawdust as a desiccant while defecating which caused the upwelling of dust while sitting, and the difficulty for children and the elderly to operate the system unassisted. By far the most important aspect that can make or break this sort of project is the presence of odour. For several reasons relating to both poor building quality and also inadequate design that did not compensate adequately for air pressure shifts inside the buildings, often persistent unacceptable odour episodes occurred. After two to three years of use, most of the households were of the opinion that the dry toilets as installed were not acceptable in the long term and further improvements would be necessary if the dry system was to be retained.

Training and management of households was also a central concern since many users tended to use the dry toilet as a solid-waste bin for disposal of disposable diapers, tampons, condoms, and even assorted packaging, plastics, and discarded clothing. Even with targeted information campaigns and demonstration, there was still a need to install a rotating cage-filter device to remove non-degradable items in the compost plant. In general, the behavioural change needed to shift to dry sanitation was a slow process for a segment of the population, while others adapted quickly. The periodic maintenance of the system such as cleaning of the urine-odour locks in the toilets was also a challenge for many households. In general, urbanites are not prepared to spend time on these sorts of household tasks and would prefer to retain a 'flush and forget' mentality. Household solid-waste management and source separation are not routinely practised in China. This hampered performance of the dry toilets and slowed the introduction of a green-bag collection programme for kitchen wastes.

The project resulted in the building of 832 apartments in 42 buildings with four and five storeys and equipping these with a complete ecosan system. All apartments were sold on the open market and the households began moving in during 2006. The ecosan system, including onsite greywater treatment plant and storage pond, was fully completed in 2007. The thermal compost plant was completed in 2008 and produced good-quality compost with elimination of pathogens in the thermal process. Large-scale demonstration of reuse was successful in potato, maize, and greenhouse vegetable gardens. The local government was not interested in reusing urine in the adjacent urban green areas due to the risk of urine odour near inhabited buildings but later on in 2009, three organic farmers were identified in order to make use of the products from the project.

The system provided continuously functioning toilets and urinals. Qualitative performance of the system did, however, experience several problems caused by various factors. These expressed themselves mainly as odour and mechanical performance of the toilet. Problems in building quality were discovered months and years after building completion. The design was not robust enough to compensate for the inherent poor building quality, poor skill level of the workers, and the overall lack of proper building and construction inspection. Users had difficulties in maintaining the dry toilets, often adding excessive amounts of water for cleaning and to reduce odour which in fact aggravated the odour problem. Additions of kitchen and solid waste to the toilets also produced odour problems. The greywater pipes were blocked for a lengthy period by soil and construction debris. Pipes were also crushed by heavy equipment and inspection wells were not sealed on the inside, allowing soil to enter the pipe system. Apartments were released to the owners before the ventilation systems were properly installed and fans were not installed on time. Urine odour vented into the toilet rooms since the outlet pipes were not immersed in the urine and vented freely back into the toilet. Hotline data showed the toilet had some technical problems and these were remedied on a case-by-case basis. Improvements were made in the ventilation system in that sealed cabinets were installed in the basements enclosing the wheelie bins.

Household responses could be categorized into three groups: a minority was very satisfied; a majority accepted the dry toilet but still hoped to have flush toilets; a minority rejected the dry ecosan system completely. In addition to the restrictions of the toilet design, an important reason for the negative attitude was the traditional culture and belief that the dry toilet is inferior to the flushed one and represents a return to rural living. The social marketing and promotion work was as effective as it could be under the circumstances of rapid urbanization and a market-based setting. To do more would entail a long-term process in terms of changing people's minds and behaviour, something that was not a part of this project.

The final work on improvement was the toilet itself. Adapting a Separett toilet with self-enclosed small-vent fan appeared to be a major improvement in ventilation performance and adapted well to the challenges around air pressure changes, in particular when households used powerful kitchen fans to evacuate cooking odours. This solution had and still has great promise but the households decided in any case to shift to a waterborne system in 2009. This 'new' system entailed using the urine tanks for sedimentation, the small-bore greywater pipe system and a simplified treatment plant. The plan was to compost the accumulated sludge along with kitchen organics. The new system is an interesting application of a sustainable sanitation system, through the use of small-bore pipes without pumps and onsite treatment with reuse of the treated products (sludge and water) and not using large sewer pipes connected to the centralized treatment plant (*ca* 10 km away).

CHAPTER 2

# Designed to close the loop

The design of the Erdos Eco-Town Project (EETP) was meant to showcase sophisticated ecological sanitation and solid waste facilities in an urban environment. The working concept behind the system design was that the separation of waste streams would increase the efficiency of treatment and facilitate the recycling process. The system design therefore focused on the separation of four main waste streams: faeces, urine, greywater, and solid waste. Each separated flow stream can be thought of as a sub-system in which the products are sanitized and recycled. For example, Figure 4 gives an overview of the systems used for collection, treatment and disposal/utilization of faeces, urine, and greywater. The toilets, urinals, and related equipment were developed and manufactured in China for this project by Chaozhou Meilong Ceramics Industry in Guangdong and are now available on the Chinese market.

Construction started at the EETP project site in July 2004. The new town was composed of 42 four- and five-storey buildings, a nursery school, a service centre, and an eco-station. Construction for the majority of the buildings was completed at the end of 2006 with 832 apartments for 3,000 residents all of which were serviced by urine-diverting toilets connected to a collection system and treatment plant at the eco-station. Construction continued into 2007 with the finalization of the greywater piping and treatment system. The eco-station in the corner of the residential area included a composting plant, solid waste station, the greywater treatment plant, and the post-treatment pond.

## Faeces system

The faeces system consisted of the toilet, a collection system of chutes and faeces bins, and finally a composting station within the eco-station. The toilet chosen for use in the EETP was a urine-diversion dry toilet which was designed to separate urine from faeces requiring no water for transporting both types of waste. The toilet design was meant to mimic a conventional toilet, complete with sawdust for 'flushing', so as to increase user familiarity and comfort. The design for the collection system used a straight-drop chute from the toilets into basement bins enclosed in cabinets. The faeces collected in these bins could then be transported to the compost station for treatment.

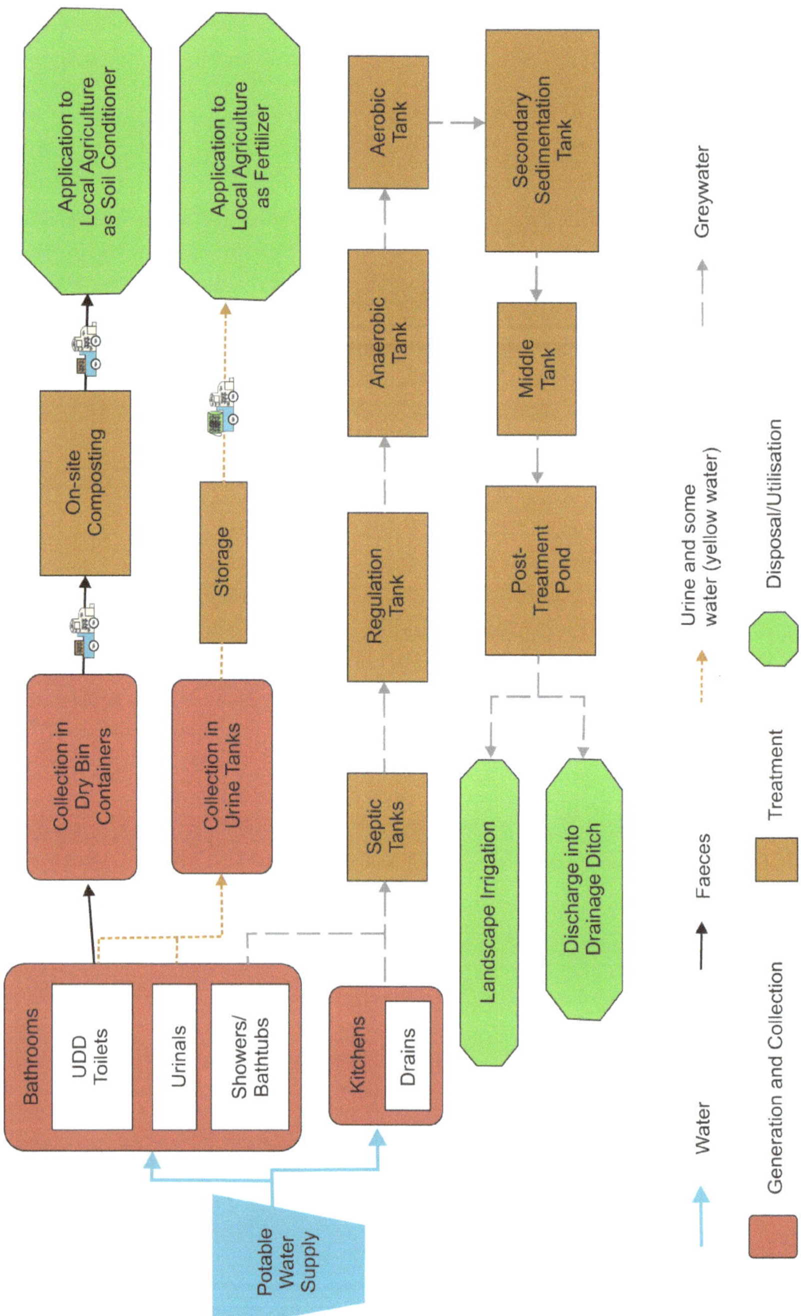


**Figure 4.** System diagram of EETP showing the flows for the faeces, urine, and greywater sub-systems
*Source:* Flores, 2010

### *Urine-diverting dry toilet*

The conceptual design for the EETP urine-diverting dry toilet (UDDT) was developed by the Swedish experts Uno Winblad and Kalle Rydberg. The basic design for the toilet consisted of two holes, with urine collected at the front of the toilet bowl and the faeces through a larger hole at the back (Figure 5). Of particular concern from the user perspective was that the toilet should seem like a modern toilet and provide a sense of cleanliness. This first porcelain model was installed in all 832 flats.

This toilet had two innovative features: a Teflon®-coated turning bowl to collect the faeces and a sawdust dispenser for 'flushing'. The purpose of the turning bowl was to avoid direct sight of faeces by the user and also to provide a safer feeling when using the toilet, especially for users on the fourth floor where there was a 12m chute to the basement. The bowl was positioned upside down when the toilet was not in use. When the user sat down, however, a lever was activated by the user's weight and rotated the bowl 180 degrees so it served as a receptacle for the faeces. The bowl fit into a steel cylinder just below the toilet bowl and was connected by a shaft to the turning mechanism (Figure 6). When the user stood up, the bowl was driven back to its standby position by a spring, and the faeces were dropped down the chute. All parts of the mechanism were made of stainless steel and the surface of both sides of the bowl and the inside of the cylinder were plated with Teflon® to reduce sticking of the faeces.

The other unique feature of this toilet was the use of sawdust for 'flushing' the faeces and absorbing odour. The sawdust also acted as an additive to the faeces to speed up the drying process. The sawdust was stored in a tank at the back of the toilet and a flushing button was used to release a fixed amount of sawdust into the bowl. Users were advised to add sawdust to the bowl before defecation to minimize sticking to the bowl's surface, and afterwards to reduce the odour from the fresh faeces. To avoid clumping of the sawdust in the tank,

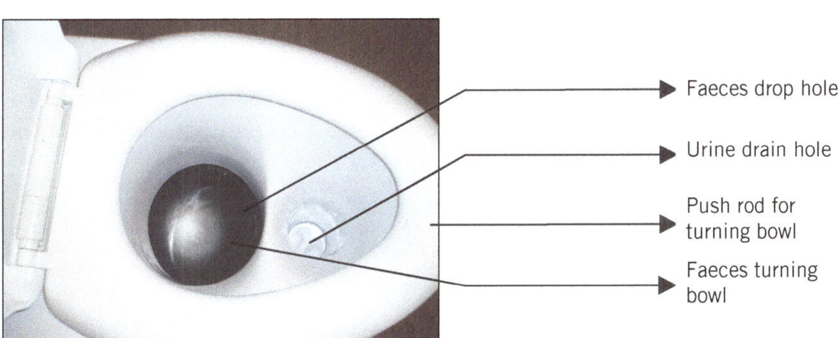


**Figure 5.** Structure of the porcelain urine-diverting dry toilet
*Source:* SEI

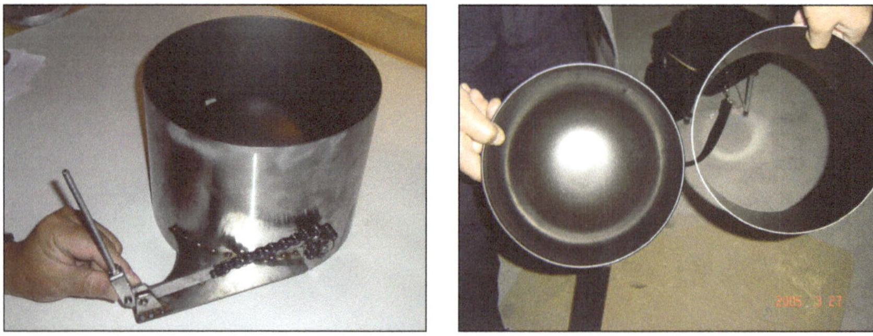

**Figure 6.** The turning mechanism and the bowl
*Source:* SEI

stirring rods that would move with each flush were attached inside the tank. The volume of the tank was designed to store sawdust for one week's use. Residents collected small bags of dried and sifted sawdust from the eco-station at no cost to them.

### *Faeces collection system*

The second step in the faeces system consisted of the chutes from the toilets, collection bins in the basement of the buildings, and transport to the eco-station. The collection system performed the intermediate steps of transport and storage of the faecal matter before it was treated at the composting plant.

*Chutes*. As shown in Figure 7, each toilet was connected to its own chute that led straight down to the collection bins below. The chutes were 280 mm diameter PVC pipes that were fixed in the floor. Toilets were placed over the chute and the turning-bowl mechanism was used to screw fast the toilet to the chute. An important design issue that should be underlined is the space requirements for having individual chutes in multi-storey buildings. Due to the chutes coming down from the upper floors, the lower floors ended up having less space available in the toilet room; for example the first floor toilet rooms were 1.6 $m^2$ smaller than those on the fourth floor.

*Collection bins*. The chutes dropped into collection bins in the basement of each apartment. The bins were commercially-available, plastic-wheeled trash bins. Each bin had a storage volume of 120 l and was designed to store the faeces from one household for at least one month. There were two basements for each stairwell, and each basement contained the bins for four to five households, depending on the number of storeys of the building. When a bin was full, the maintenance team removed it and replaced it with an empty one.

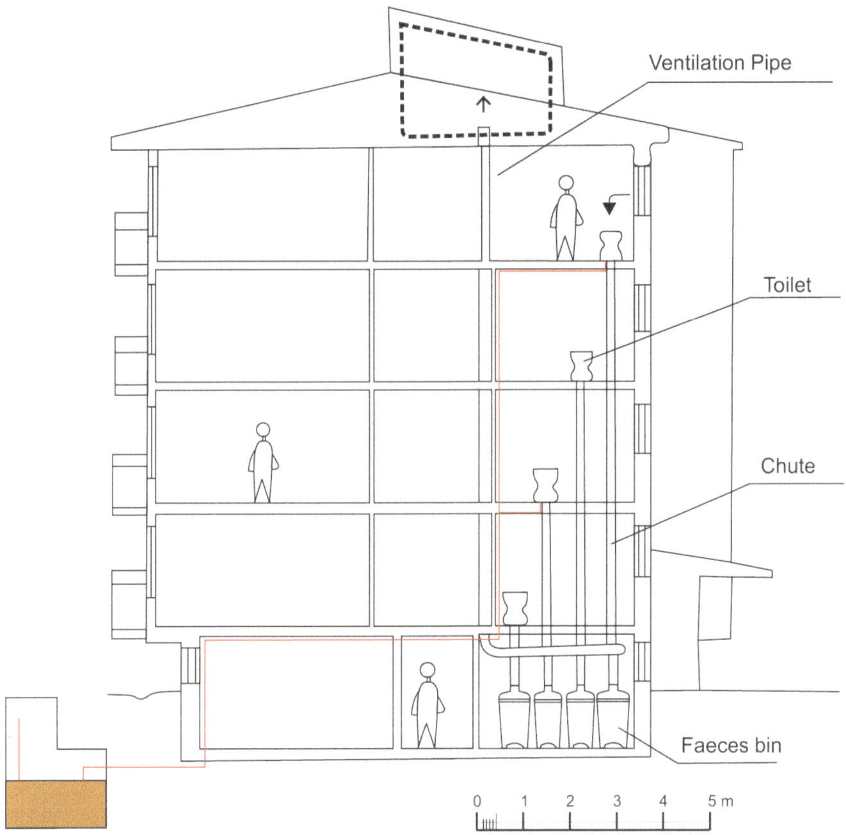


**Figure 7.** Illustration of the faeces and urine system

In order to prevent bad odours in the basement, the bins needed to be covered and vented. The original design used a movable sealed cover, which was fixed on the back wall of the basement (Figure 8). The lids were made of PVC and connected by a steel lifting mechanism to the wall. There were two holes in the lid, one for the chute and the other for the vent pipe. The seal between the lid and bin was made from 5 cm thick plastic foam. In this model the cover was lifted off when the bin needed to be removed and then lowered back onto the emptied bin when it was put back in place. This model was designed to save space in the basement and provide for easy removal of the covers during maintenance.

Since it was attached to the wall, however, the cover required that bins were positioned correctly for them to seal properly. This meant that more care needed to be taken by the maintenance team during the emptying process. The problem was exacerbated by construction errors in the alignment of the

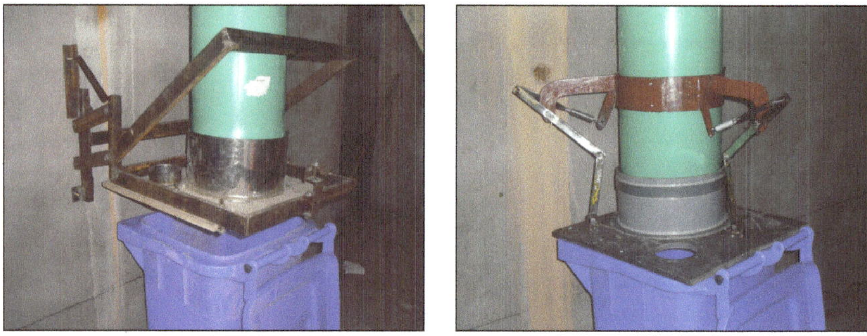

**Figure 8.** Two models of the initial lifting mechanism for the bin covers: original model attached to the wall (left) and the adaptation to connect it directly to the chute (right)
*Source:* SEI

chutes and bin covers. Positioning of the chute during construction was often 3–5 cm off-centre, which made it difficult to install the bin covers properly. In some cases the error was even greater and the bin covers would not fit at all. In order to correct this problem, the lifting mechanism was redesigned to fit around the chute itself instead of to the wall (Figure 8b). A lever and spring system lifted the lid and also applied pressure on the lid to form a tight seal.

*Basement access.* Access for removal and maintenance of the bins was an important design consideration. The bins needed to be taken out of the basements regularly and replaced with empty ones. Originally, multiple basements in each building were designed to be connected by corridors with ramps leading to the outside of the building. This design was found to be too material-intensive and expensive, aesthetically-displeasing, and sometimes physically impossible due to slope and space considerations for construction of the ramps. The compromise involved removing the corridors and providing separate access to each basement via an external access pit, similar to a cellar. In some cases when two basements were adjacent to each other, they were connected with a short corridor and had the same access pit. Bins were removed via the basements from the access pit by using a simple hoist installed on a light truck. The truck then transported the bins to the composting plant.

### *Ventilation system*

An important part of the faeces system was the ventilation system to mitigate odours from the faecal bins. The system was designed so that foul air from the toilets and collection bins was directed to a vent pipe on the roof, thereby eliminating odour problems in the household (Figure 9). Airflow in the system moved down the chute from the toilet room, through the bins, into the ventilation pipes, and out through the vent pipe on the roof. A fan in the

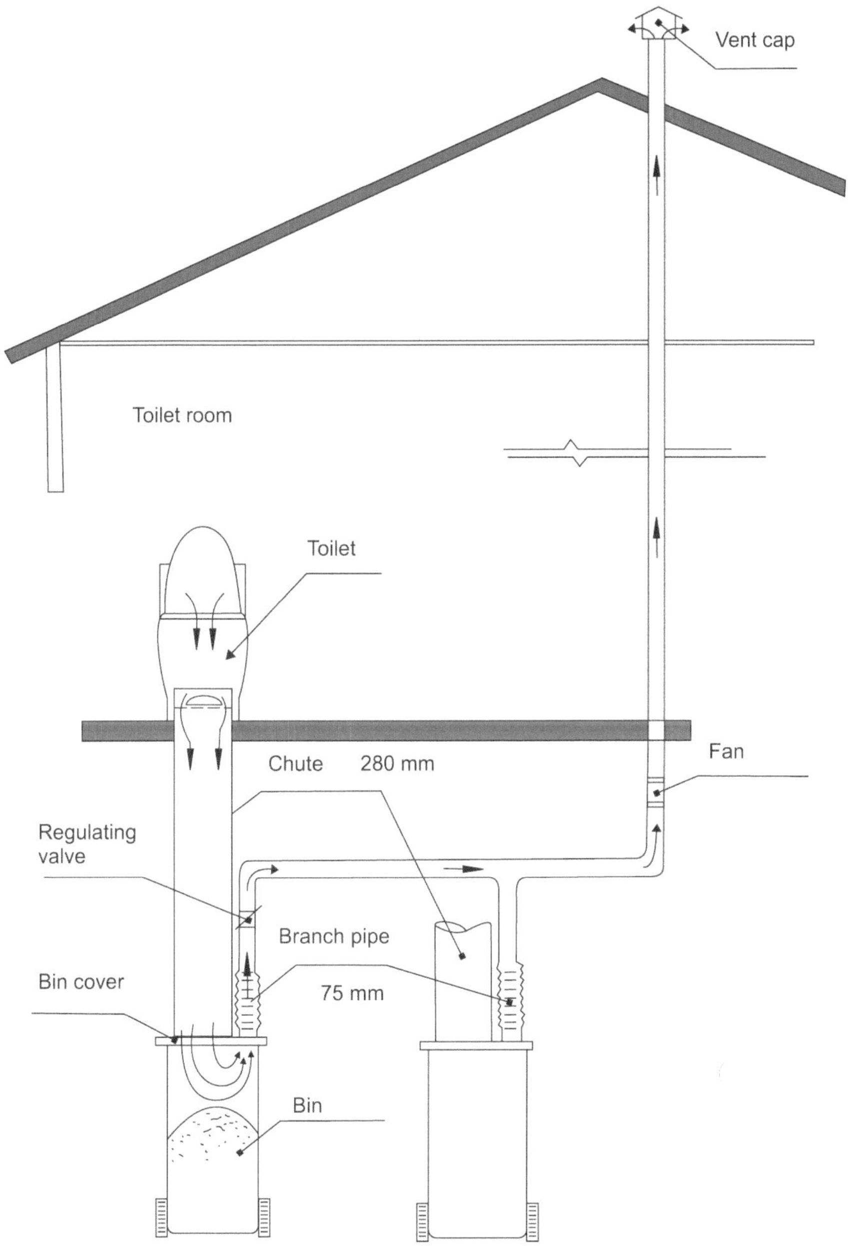


**Figure 9.** Ventilation system showing the toilet, drop chute, collector bin, fan, vent pipe, and vent-pipe cap

basement vent pipe drove the airflow. The ventilation system was designed according to recommended standards for heating and ventilation, which would change the air in the toilet room every 40 minutes; moving approximately 30 $m^3$ of air per hour. Based on airflow calculations and the capacity of fans available on the market it was determined that one axial fan in each basement would be sufficient for four to five toilets.

### *Compost plant*

The original idea for the composting plant was to do indoor composting in windrows. The building would be kept simple with a cement floor to make turning easier and the air inside would be deodorized before it was released to the outside using water filtration. Workers were not trained in composting techniques, however, and additional organic matter and soil was not available to mix with the faeces when the plant started operation in January 2007. When the first two pick-up trucks of bins containing the faeces were brought to the plant, the contents were simply dumped on the floor, creating a smelly mess. The odour was unacceptable and created a very negative first impression of the compost plant. The DPO called off work at the indoor plant for the rest of the year and faeces were taken to a farm 10 km away for outdoor composting.

A second attempt at an indoor composting machine was developed by the Beijing Agriculture University in 2007. The machine prototype was reported to process organic waste, animal manure, and human waste within 15 days. Performance requirements for the procured composting machine included a stainless steel composting bin, sharp razor edges to break down plastics in the raw material, and the ability to monitor temperature and humidity (Zhu, 2008). The machine was tested in 2007, but did not drain properly and could not handle the large volumes of solid waste that ended up in the faecal bins.

Finally, Lvhuanben Science & Technology Co. Ltd. was commissioned to design an indoor composting facility. The composting plant was based on common Chinese design with batch-aerated composting chambers (each 6$m^3$) and seeding with micro-organisms to accelerate the decomposition process. The system was partly mechanized and partly manual labour to process the estimated 1,200 kg/day of faeces and organic kitchen waste that was generated at the EETP. The running costs were expected to be low and the system easy to maintain and control. According to the design consultant, the compost procedure had been tried in small scale and samples of the resulting compost indicated that it could meet the criteria for organic fertilizer stipulated in the national code. The machine from Beiing Agriculture University was converted into the pre-compost mixer and screening device for the removal of solid waste (plastic bags, diapers, bottles, etc).

The composting plant was designed to minimize public health risks from the use of composted faeces for agriculture. The World Health Organization (WHO) has guidelines for the safe reuse of faecal material in agriculture application (WHO, 2006: 63) which recommend 'thermophilic digestion

(50°C for 14 days) and composting in aerated piles for one month at 55–60°C' as generally accepted procedure for treatment of human excreta. The WHO report refers to the work of Haug (1993), which showed that, 'under controlled conditions, composting at 55–60°C for one to two days is sufficient to kill essentially all pathogens'; the longer recommended processing periods are intended to provide a safety margin related to the handling of the faecal materials. A properly functioning thermophilic composting system requires not only moisture and aeration, but also a good carbon-to-nitrogen ratio in the compost materials. As the microorganisms digest and transform the organic matter in the compost materials, they grow and multiply using the carbon and nitrogen as building blocks for their cells at a ratio of 30 parts carbon (C) to 1 part nitrogen (N). Excess nitrogen gets converted to ammonia, causing odours (Jenkins, 2005). Esrey *et al.* (1998) therefore recommends a C:N ratio of between 15:1 and 30:1, while Jenkins (2005) recommends a ratio between 20:1 and 35:1. Human faeces has a C:N ratio of 5:10 (Jenkins, 2005), and will therefore not compost properly by itself. At the EETP, sawdust was added to absorb moisture and increase the carbon content of the compost materials. Raw sawdust contains very little nitrogen relative to faeces and is approximately 50 per cent carbon (Jenkins, 2005). Kitchen organic matter was intended to be composted with the faeces, so as to help achieve the right C:N ratio.

The composting process started by emptying the faecal matter into the mixing machine for removal of the solid waste that ended up in the collection bins. Afterwards the organic matter was mechanically mixed with additional sawdust to arrive at the optimal level of humidity and inoculated with a mixture of 'effective micro-organisms' to facilitate degradation of organic matter. Then the material was manually placed in one of the six composting chambers. The composting process was designed in two steps. First was an aerobic phase during which the temperature in the composting pile would reach 70°C for a period of four to five days in order to reduce pathogen concentrations to safe levels (Zhu, 2008). Following the aerobic phase, the material would be transferred to another chamber for a fermenting period of 25–30 days. During the fermenting stage, the compost was heated but not aerated. The chambers were aerated by pumping air through small openings in the cement floor and heated using electrical cables under the floor. The plant was designed for solar heating during winter with supplementary heat from a coal-fired stove during extremely cold periods. The entire composting cycle was 35 days. At the end of the process the finished fertilizer product was packaged in bags for later transport and reuse. Quality control and analysis of bacterial and nutrient content were carried out as part of the R&D of the project.

## Urine system

Diversion of urine is the most efficient way to maximize reuse of the nutrients in human excreta and urine contains the majority of the nutrients leaving the body (Vinnerås *et al.*, 2006). Although urine is generally sterile, it can contain some pathogens, especially if the system is misused and faecal matter or greywater mixes with the urine. Sterilization of urine is achieved through storage in a closed container where the elevated pH caused by the ammonia content will cause pathogen die-off. Storage time is temperature-dependent and can also be affected by dilution of the urine (WHO, 2006). Afterwards, the sterile liquid can be applied to agriculture as a fertilizer. Although treatment of urine is relatively simple, it is also the fraction of excreta that causes the most odour (ammonia gas). Therefore, odour control is an important aspect of a urine-diverting and storage system.

### *Urine collection*

Urine was collected from the urinals and the UDDTs. Each toilet room was fitted with a toilet and a urinal which both emptied into the urine-piping system and eventually to the storage tanks. Urine from the toilet was collected through the hole at the front of the toilet bowl (Figure 5). The original toilet

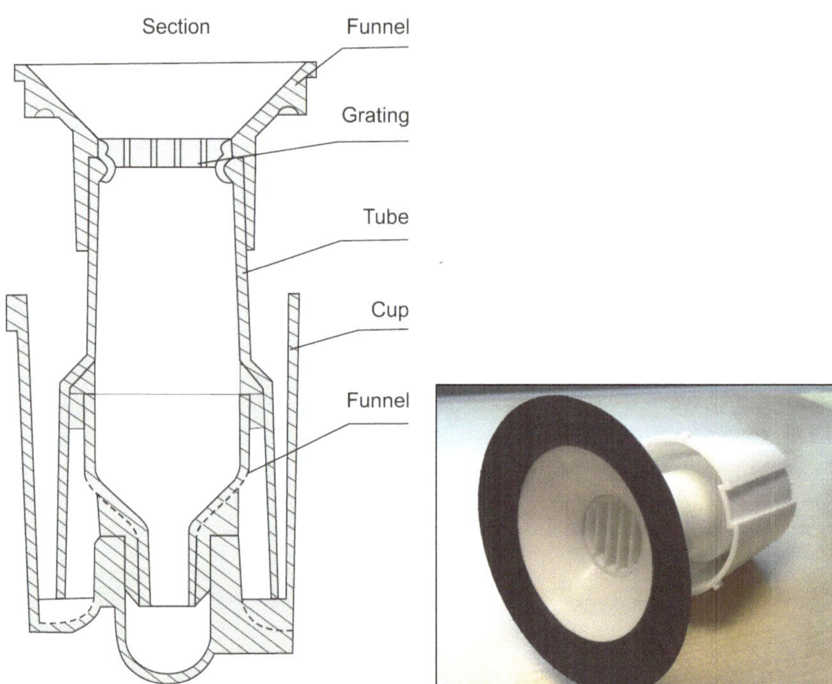


**Figure 10.** Cross-section and photograph of the urine-odour trap placed in the porcelain toilet designed to include a thin layer of paraffin oil to help seal the urine from the atmosphere. Manufactured by Xindahua Plastic Industrial Co Ltd, Chaozhou, Guangdong Prov, China
*Source:* Courtesy of Karl Rydberg©

design included a perforated, circular, porcelain plate over the hole to inhibit odour and allow for drainage. This design was insufficient at controlling the smell of urine in the toilet room, so a new odour trap was introduced which contained a layer of paraffin oil that floated on top of the urine captured in the trap, thereby preventing the escape of odour-causing gases from the urine hole (Figure 10). Maintenance of the odour trap required periodic addition of paraffin oil to replace that which was lost during repeated use and cleaning.

Initially, there was no odour control mechanism connected to the urinal, just a straight pipe connected to the urine piping system. During use of the system, however, it was found that there were problems with odour coming up from the urinal pipes, so a standard 'S' trap was installed to mitigate the problem. The 'S' trap was made from plastic material to avoid corrosion by the hydrochloric acid used for cleaning the urine crystal adhered to the wall of the trap. Unfortunately, this only partially solved the problem. Since the urinals were designed to use a minimal amount of water for cleaning, the trap was often filled with a mixture of urine and water, resulting in odour. The installation of larger urinals with odour traps similar to the ones installed in the toilets was discussed but never implemented.

The urine collected from the toilets and urinals flowed into the urine pipe system. This system was arranged similarly to conventional wastewater pipes in multi-storey buildings. Pipes from each floor were connected to a main pipe in the basement which was linked to a trunk pipe leading to a storage tank. The urine pipe system was semi-centralized with one tank serving two to three buildings. Pipeline segments were designed to be less than 200 m in length to avoid precipitation on the pipe walls and blockages. The underground pipelines carrying urine from the toilets to the storage tanks were designed to be buried below the frost line of 1.5 m; however, due to construction error, most of the pipelines were buried at 1.2 m. Segments of pipelines consequently froze in the winter and had to be replaced. The pipes in the basements were subsequently insulated as well.

### *Urine storage tanks*

Dimensioning of the urine storage tanks was based on a monthly emptying schedule and an estimated urine production of 360 l/person/yr. Based on these calculations, a total of 22 tanks were installed, varying from 5 to 13.5 $m^3$ in volume. The tanks were buried to avoid freezing during the winter. The tank design required that the inlet pipe to the tanks be submerged to stop ammonia gas from being vented back up the urine pipes and into the toilet rooms. A bucket was therefore placed under each inlet pipe to ensure that, even with minimal flow into the tank, the inlet pipe would remain submerged below liquid level.

The urine tanks were sealed with reinforced concrete covers to prevent the loss of nitrogen during storage, to protect the tank, and to prevent dirt from dropping into the tank. Emptying of the tanks was done by a suction truck that accessed the tanks via quick-coupling valves set into the covers. The truck would then transport the urine directly to a local farmer for storage before application to the fields.

## Greywater system

The household greywater from sinks and showers in the EETP was managed separately from the human excreta. Although there were several options for treatmeant of greywater, the result of the planning discussions was the adoption of a conventional, bio-filtering technique. The system included a pre-treatment tank for sedimentation followed by an aerobic treatment plant to remove organics and finally a post-treatment pond for final polishing. The design for the system was carried out by Tianjin Academy of Environment Science (TAES) in China.

### *Greywater piping system*

The piping system to collect household greywater was designed on the same concept as the urine system. Greywater from individual households was piped to a larger branch pipe that collected the flow from four households before connecting to the trunk pipe. The pipe system was designed to ensure a slope that was not less than 0.5 per cent so as to prevent solid deposition and blockage, at the same time as it was buried deep enough to be below the frost-depth. Due to topographical constraints, the pipe system was divided into two lines, east and west. The east line collected from 12 buildings and the west line from the remaining 31 buildings. The two lines met at a well located just before the septic tank at the start of the greywater treatment system.

Besides the pipes, the greywater system included odour-management devices and access points for maintenance. At the household level, the greywater pipes had a water lock in the shower drain to prevent odour from returning up the pipe system. In addition, ventilation pipes for each of the branch pipes extended above the roof. Inspection wells for maintenance access were also installed at key points in the underground trunk system. The covers of the inspection wells were originally designed to be airtight to avoid odour problems, but such models were not available on the local market, so conventional cast-iron lids were used instead. Unfortunately, some of the inspection wells remained without covers until late 2006, and were used for dumping household solid waste. This created blockages within the system and the estate management staff had to regularly clean the wells to maintain flow in the system.

In addition to problems with open manholes, the piping system initially ran into trouble with hydraulic flow in the pipes. Many of the pipes were originally installed at elevations higher than what was specified in the design. The result was that many sections of pipe froze during the winter of 2005–2006, and/or experienced clogging as the result of low hydraulic head. In addition, many of the pipes were damaged by heavy machinery during construction of the buildings, resulting in blocked pipes or leakages. As a result, the discharge into the treatment plant prior to 2006 was so low that the plant could not be operated. In 2006, a number of pipes were re-laid so that they were below the frost-depth and deep enough to improve the hydraulic flow. By the end of May 2007, all the obstructions in the pipes had been cleared and the greywater plant became fully operational.

### *Treatment of greywater*

The treatment plant was designed to treat the greywater produced by the 832 households in the Erdos sub-division. The most important design criteria for the treatment plant were the amount of water to be treated and the effluent quality guidelines. Greywater generation was calculated from expected water consumption habits and the number of inhabitants. In Inner Mongolia and northern China water supply is estimated at 120 l/person/day; however, given a dry system without flushing water in the toilet, water savings of 30 l/person/day were expected. Considering that some water would be lost due to urine diversion, or during other household uses, the predicted greywater production was 80 l/person/day. Given that the average family size in Dongsheng was 3.5, the treatment capacity of the plant needed to be 250 $m^3$/day.

The plant was designed to meet two levels of treatment standards: the National Code for Grade II Effluent and the National Code for Reclaimed Water for Miscellaneous Use. The Dongsheng District is regulated under Grade II standards, which apply to discharges into water bodies for general industrial water supply, recreational waters in which there is no direct human contact with the water, and water bodies for agricultural water supply and for general landscape requirements. Meeting requirements for reclaimed water would mean even greater water savings as water could be reused within the eco-town for landscape irrigation. There was no information available in China about pollution loads and typical characteristics of greywater, therefore it was estimated that the incoming water to the plant would be similar to typical loading values found in the literature. It was later found that the pollutant concentration of raw greywater was greatly underestimated, due to the low volumes of water used by the households which made the greywater chemical oxidation demand (COD) content more concentrated.

The greywater treatment plant recommended by TAES was mainly an aerobic process (biofilm oxidation),with an anaerobic process added to enable the system to meet the National Code for Grade II effluent. The raw greywater first flowed into a septic tank fitted with a grease trap for pre-settlement and initial anaerobic treatment (Figure 11). From there the water flowed into a buffer tank that assured uniform water quality and quantity before flowing into the oxidation chamber. These treatment processes were followed by a secondary sedimentation tank to separate the liquids and solids. Finally, the water flowed into the transition tank before moving to the post-treatment

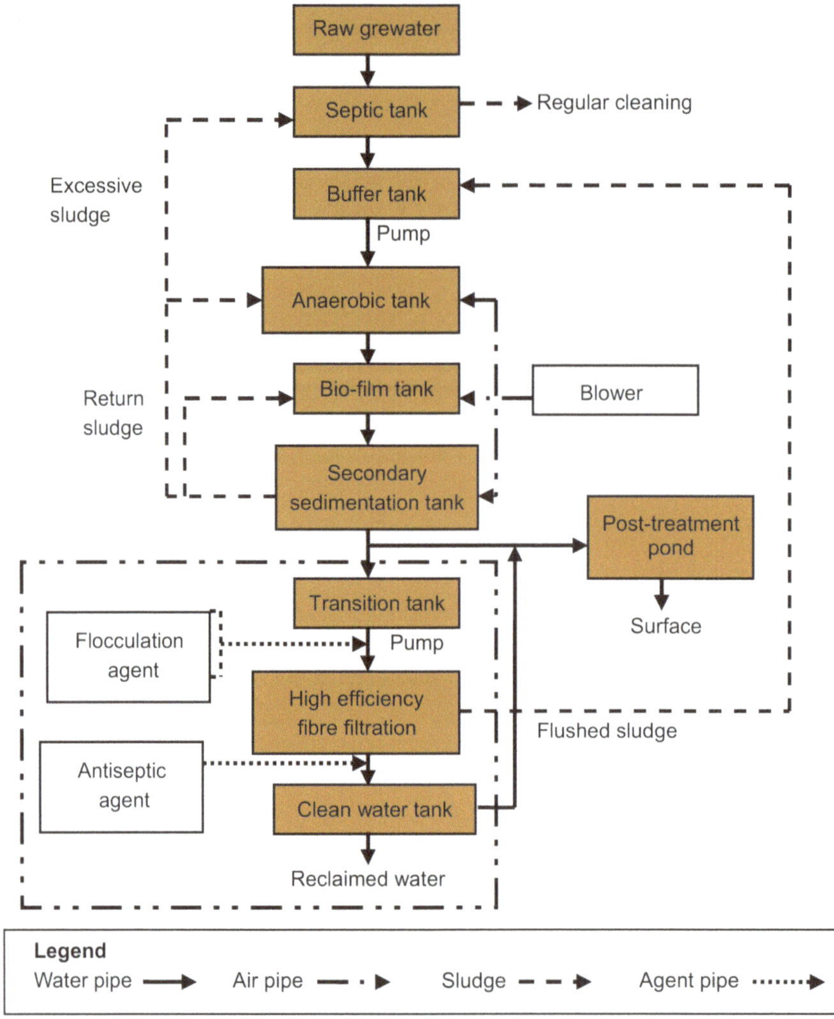


**Figure 11.** Flow chart of the greywater treatment system
*Source:* Courtesy of Tianjin Academy of Environmental Sciences

pond or for treatment to reclaimed water standards. Treatment to reach reclaimed water quality standards was achieved in an additional step, during which chemical agents were added and the water filtered through a high-efficiency fibre filter before sterilization. The reclaimed water was stored in a cistern as a supply for local urban irrigation. Water that was not treated to reclaimed water quality was emptied into the post-treatment pond.

### *Post-treatment pond*

The pond was designed for use as a storage tank and final polishing step in the treatment process, before the water drained to a nearby stream. In addition to treatment, it was hoped that the pond would add to the aesthetics of the area. The post-treatment pond was located in a depression near the eco-station in the north-west corner of the project area. The location of the pond was chosen to take advantage of the low elevation and its distance away from the housing area, since the local authorities were worried about odour. The pond was bound by roads to the north and west, and by a footpath to the east. The eco-station and composting plant were located on the south side of the pond.

In designing the pond, two key requirements were taken into consideration: (1) that the pond should be deep enough to ensure flow of water below the ice in the winter; and (2) that it could accommodate heavy storm-water flow in case of a flood. During the winter months it was determined that the pond depth should be kept at a maximum to avoid it freezing solid. Based on normal meteorological conditions it was estimated that a maximum water depth of 1.8 m would be adequate to prevent blockage of the inlet pipe by ice. Therefore, given the topography of the existing depression the surface area and storage volume of the pond were calculated to be 3,670 $m^2$ and 3,700 $m^3$, respectively. In order to address the second concern, it was determined that it was necessary to add a sluice for storm-water drainage. An extra outlet for storm-water drainage was added on the north side of the pond, which emptied through a culvert under the road to a drainage ditch. The sluice was fitted with a manually controlled sluice gate to regulate the flow (Figure 12).

The basic design of the treatment pond consisted of dykes around the entire depression area, inlet pipes, an outlet pipe for treated water, and the sluice with a storm outlet. The concrete slab dykes were insulated with polypropylene foam to prevent damage from frost in the winter. The two dykes that bordered the roads were also lined with a geo-membrane to prevent water seepage under the roadbed that could damage the road foundations. The south and east dykes were not made watertight so that aquatic plants could be planted along the shores, adding to the nutrient-absorbing capacity of the pond and improving aesthetics. The outlet pipe from the pond emptied through a 315 m-long pipe under the highway to the west where it discharged into an open ditch. The discharge essentially functioned as a groundwater infiltration source and evapo-transpiration system.

## Solid waste system

The final waste stream to be managed by the eco-town project was household solid waste. The original project plan was to adapt source-separation models used in some Swedish municipalities to Chinese conditions and test their feasibility. The organic and non-organic fractions of the household waste would be separated, preferably by the households themselves. The organic

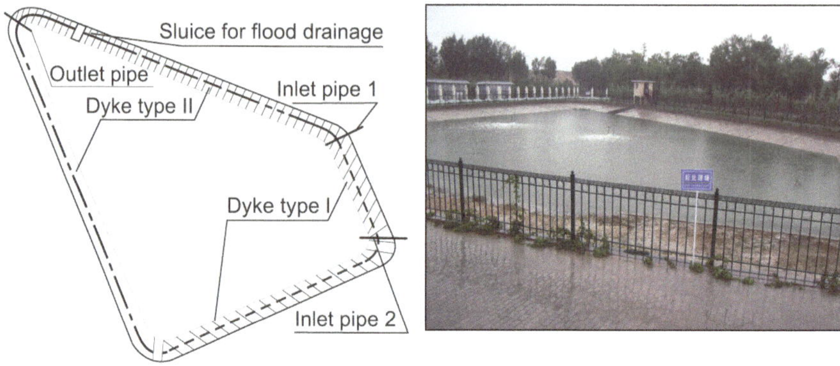


**Figure 12.** The post-treatment holding pond for greywater
*Source:* SEI

fraction could then be composted onsite with the faeces, while the non-organic waste could be sent to the municipal solid waste treatment plant for further recycling or landfilling. Implementing this type of system would require a sustained awareness-raising campaign to promote source separation in all households and places of work. The source-separating campaign did not start until autumn of 2009 when the dry-toilet system had already been changed to mini-flush toilets. This aspect did not have sufficient time to mature enough to be part of the original project and is therefore not covered in this book. The experience from the project showed that source-separation by households, especially of organic fractions, is something that is relatively new in China and not something that households were interested in carrying out. In fact, there was a common practice of throwing all solid waste into the dry toilet which created considerable problems in the composting step. A special rotating cage was necessary to remove the solid waste prior to composting. It is of interest to note that the city of Dongsheng that same year installed a centralized solid-waste plant designed to produce biogas from household wastes and a dried pelletized fertilizer from the remaining sludge.

CHAPTER 3

# Operations and maintenance

## Organization

Management of the operations and maintenance (O&M) of the EETP sanitation system was jointly controlled by the SPO and the DPO (Figure 13). The two management teams were responsible for the logistics and running of the project office. The office was initially located downtown in one of the municipal government buildings; however, in 2007, it was moved to

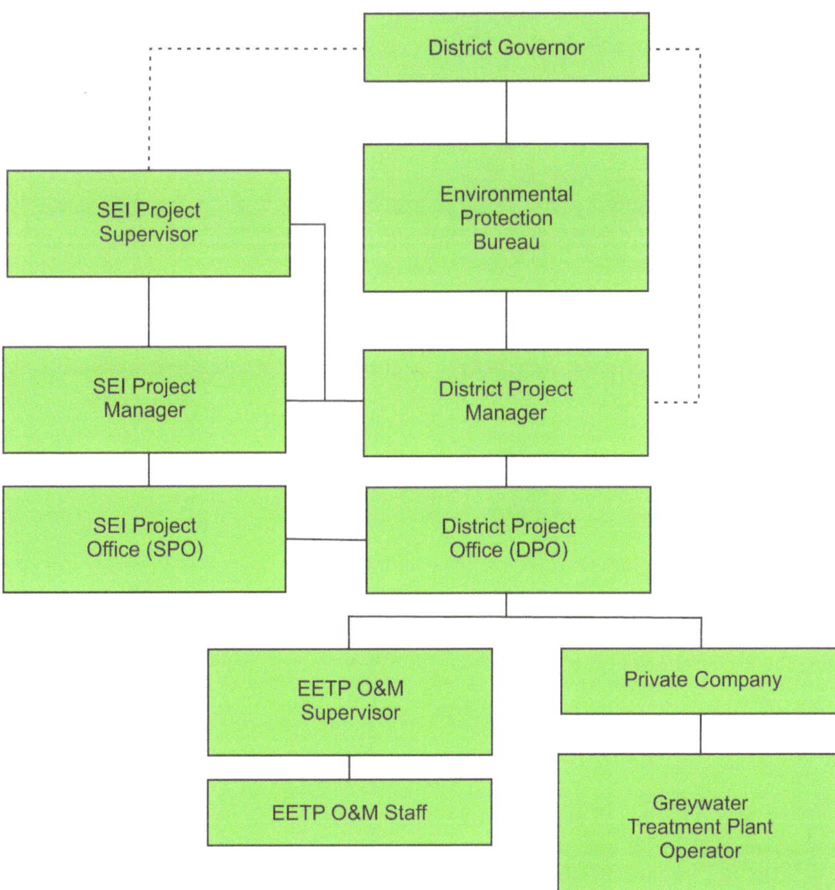


**Figure 13.** Management structure for the Erdos Eco-Town Project

the new eco-station building when it was completed on-site. In addition to management staff, the project office also housed the maintenance team and hotline service that was in charge of day-to-day operations.

*Project offices.* The SPO consisted of two to three staff members that were in charge of reporting, communication, purchasing, and day-to-day management. The SPO communicated closely with the SEI project supervisor in Stockholm and with the DPO. The SPO provided technical expertise while the DPO performed financial management for the Chinese side of the project and provided input to the periodic project reporting to SEI. The DPO lacked technical expertise and also lacked the power to intervene with the building company. That power rested with the District Governor.

*Maintenance team.* Since all these facilities were onsite, the eco-town had its own maintenance team that was responsible for operating and maintaining the system. The team was set up under the Dongsheng Project Office (DPO) in January 2006. The maintenance team consisted of eight workers and a crew leader responsible for coordinating the activities of the team. The maintenance work was paid for by the DPO and SPO.

In general, the maintenance team was in charge of the daily operations of the entire sanitation system. They were also responsible for responding to complaints from the households and assisting with user education. The maintenance team was responsible for operating the compost treatment plant, however operation of the greywater treatment plant was contracted out. The maintenance team was in charge of cleaning the basements, emptying and carrying the bins, and maintaining/repairing the toilets. The team was divided into two groups: six workers focused on servicing the households and four others were trained to manage the compost plant, although they also responded to household calls. All the workers were involved in maintenance of the basements. They worked six days a week and split the weekend shifts so that there were four workers on Saturday and Sunday.

## Household level

As with any sanitation technology, the dry toilet demanded a certain amount of maintenance effort from the households to keep it clean and functional. Although the toilet installed in the eco-town was designed to resemble a modern porcelain toilet, complete with a mechanical flush, there were a number of different rules that had to be followed. Above all, as a dry toilet it was essential that the contents of the faecal bins under the toilets be kept as dry as possible. Excess water in the faecal system not only made the treatment process more difficult, but also increased odour, something that directly affected the users' experience with the toilet. Therefore, two key maintenance issues that needed to be addressed at the household level were awareness of how the system worked and proper cleaning procedures that satisfied user hygiene standards and kept the system dry.

## *User education*

The UDDT was a new experience for the residents moving into the eco-town. The majority of them had flush toilets in their previous homes or used Chinese public toilets (flush or traditional pits). Training and education about the system was therefore necessary to teach residents how to properly use and appreciate their new toilet. The users received brochures and promotional information regarding the toilet (Figure 14) and were invited to visit the exhibit hall in the centrally-located commercial building.

There were two main issues related to user education, namely promotion of correct usage and persuasion surrounding the benefits of the dry system. The first was needed since none of the users had previous experience with a sawdust-flushing dry toilet. The second was necessary because initial surveys of the community showed that a majority of them preferred water-flush toilets. It was hoped, however, that they could be persuaded to join the minority opinion that dry toilets could be convenient and flexible in a city known for water rationing. The DPO therefore established a promotional social-work team to work with user education.

The need for a promotional and community expert was identified in the project document as early as 2004. The job description for this expert included developing information packages and training for residents, including the concept of a closed-loop system and general news updates specific to the EETP. The community worker was to be available to answer questions from residents and communicate with local officials and the media. In 2006, the SPO hired a middle-aged woman, a retired political consultant, as the EETP social worker in charge of addressing educational and behavioural-change issues surrounding the dry-sanitation system. She was supported in her work by the maintenance staff of the eco-station.

The original plan was that each household would be provided with instructions on how to use the dry toilets and urinals correctly when they moved into their flat. Due to a lack of time and communication between the developer who was in charge of selling the apartments and the project offices, however, many residents moved in without receiving proper training on the use of their new toilet.

Towards the end of 2006, the social worker, with the support of the maintenance team, began the first of three promotion periods. The promotional work was divided into three main tasks: door-to-door visits, prolonged one-on-one interviews, and specified promotion for the elderly, disabled, or temporary residents. In cases of recurring problems, the staff arranged for follow-up visits or telephone communication. For nine months during 2006–2007, the team put significant effort into increasing the acceptance of the dry toilets by visiting households directly addressing technical problems

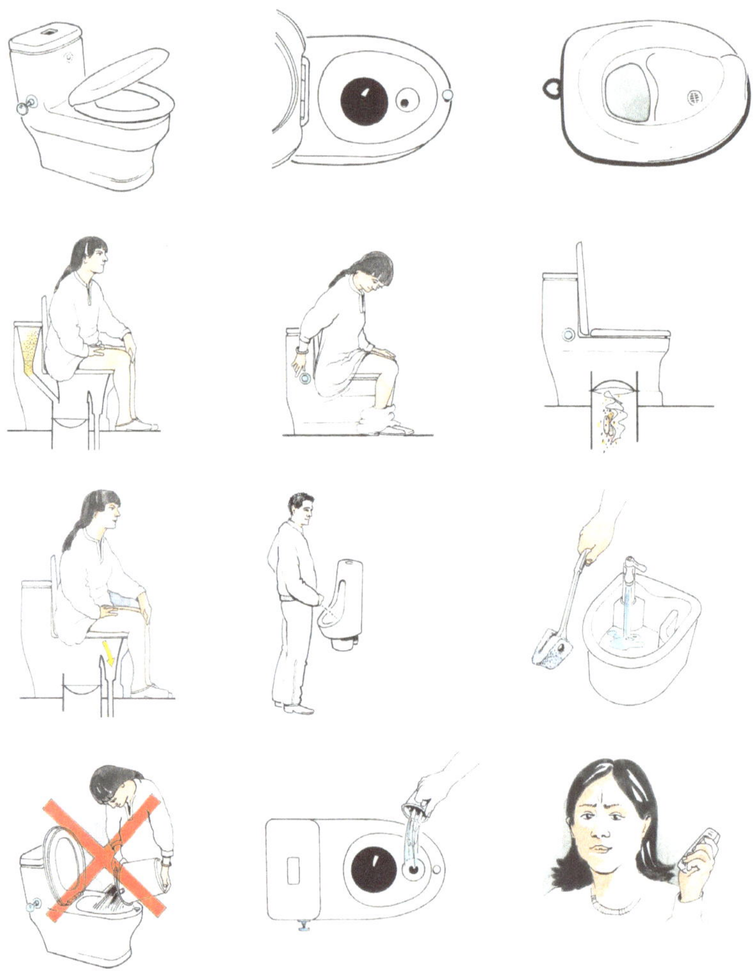

**Figure 14.** Graphics from the instruction poster on use of the urine-diverting dry toilet and urinal, distributed and explained to each household along with the hotline telephone information

they were having, explaining how the system worked, and providing training as necessary. They did door-to-door promotion with 385 apartments (Lingna, 2007), as well as specific visits with problem households or strongly dissatisfied owners. Problem households were ones which regularly poured too much water down their toilets to clean them or used them to dispose of other solid waste. Of course, the excess water in the system caused or worsened the odour problems and therefore many of these problem households were also highly dissatisfied. The social worker and members of the maintenance team met with these residents on a one-on-one basis approximately twice a week over several months, discussing their complaints and possible solutions, and reviewing the operation and maintenance procedures with them. At the end of this period, they found that problem households had been reduced from 96 to 39 apartments.

### *Cleaning*

Households were responsible for cleaning and basic maintenance of the toilets. The main challenges of the dry toilets from the household perspective included proper diversion of urine and faeces in the toilet bowl, keeping the toilet clean while minimizing the use of water and chemicals, and the presence of odour (Lingna, 2007). Of course, these problems are inter-related, as incorrect usage of the toilet receptacles or strong odour motivated people to clean the toilet and the natural tendency was to use soap and water which only worsened the problem. At the beginning of their work, the promotional team found that more than half of the households were using the toilets incorrectly by putting too much water into the system.

The majority of households reported that they cleaned the toilet several times (two to three) a week and some people did it as often as every day (Flores, 2010). Adapting to new cleaning methods presented a major challenge to many users since they had previously been used to using soap and water for toilet cleaning – something which was forbidden with the dry toilet. There were many problems in the beginning with odour caused by excess water in the collection bins. The maintenance team, therefore, invented the 'Dry Wash Method' for cleaning the toilets. This method cleaned the toilet with a special brush covered in sawdust. First, the brush was dipped in a little bit of water and then dipped in sawdust. In this way, the toilet could be cleaned, at the same time making sure that almost no water reached the faeces bin. Training in this cleaning method became part of the door-to-door campaign of the promotional team and the instruction manual that was circulated to the households.

The cleaning method introduced by the promotional team was generally adopted by the users and reports from the maintenance team showed that the number of problem households dropped over time. A survey done in spring of 2009 found that a majority of households cleaned the toilet with a brush and some water, although there were still many that used only water cleaning. Some households also used towels, cleansing agents or just sawdust for cleaning. A large majority of respondents, however, found that cleaning was troublesome. The trouble with cleaning the bowl was that the faecal matter and sawdust would often dry on the bowl, requiring hard scrubbing to get it clean. The shape and positioning of the turning bowl also meant that it was hard to reach all sides of the bowl. It was necessary to push down on the seat while cleaning to turn the bowl into the proper position. Many households who had had flush toilets before reported that they found cleaning much easier with a water-flushed bowl.

In addition to cleaning the toilet, the use of sawdust in the toilet created extra maintenance work and worries for some users. There were problems with sawdust building up in the faecal chute and eventually clogging it so that users had to push on the solidified mass from the edges of the chute to get it to fall down. Others complained about the dust escaping the toilet bowl into the rest of the room during use and operation of the sawdust dispenser. This made for extra cleaning in the toilet room as the sawdust accumulated in the cracks and corners. In addition, some people were worried about potential health consequences from bacterial contamination in the sawdust, especially for women when they are seated on the toilet. There were some reports (unconfirmed) of women contracting genital irritation from using the toilets with sawdust.

The most significant complaint related to household maintenance was the presence of odour from the toilets, the urine system, and greywater drains. In general, odour from the faecal bins was minimized if they were kept dry. There were other technical problems with the ventilation system that led to odour problems for some residents, especially those on the top floors. Household-level problems in the urine system were mainly related to the odour traps in the toilets and urinals. The urine-odour traps required occasional cleaning to remove the build up of scale within the pipe. Households were recommended to regularly clean the odour traps; the majority of households preferred to call the maintenance team to clean or replace them. It was obvious that there was some frustration related to the cleaning of the traps, or perhaps a lack of understanding, since many odour traps were thrown down the faecal chutes to be taken away with the faeces. In 2008, a waterless trap, the 'Dry Smell Stop' was tested in several households which seemed to improve the situation.

Aside from the odour traps, the urinals also created some problems at the household level. Many men discovered that the size of the urinal was too small and/or installed too low, so that urine often splashed out to the floor. This created a mess and added to the unpleasant smells in the toilet room. Several residents reported that the position of the urinals was more appropriate for children than for adult males.

To some degree, household maintenance could also affect the level of odour coming from the floor drains for the greywater system. The locally available water-lock was very small and the water quickly evaporated, releasing a bad smell. The problem was exacerbated by the in-floor heating system in the apartments (first of its kind in the area) that increased the evaporation rate. Households could fix the problem by adding more water to the water-lock, however this often had to be done every few hours. The maintenance team would inform households to cover floor drains tightly when not in use, and frequently recharge the odour-lock with water, however this advice was not always followed.

### *Maintenance hotline for homeowners*

At the household level, the residents were supported by the project maintenance team. A telephone hotline was established at the eco-station so that households could report problems with their toilets. A receptionist was hired to answer the hotline during the working week. During evenings and weekends, the calls were transferred to the maintenance workers' cell phones. In this way the hotline was always open since there were workers onsite seven days a week, including night duty. The complaints were recorded on a database and a worker was dispatched to fix the problem. Response time was under 30 minutes, and often within five minutes. Unless spare parts were lacking, the repair work would be completed within the same day.

When called, a member of the maintenance team would arrive at the household armed with protective clothing, safety gloves, rubber boots, and a tool box full of items for repairing and cleaning (e.g. handsaw, forceps, silicone, screwdriver, brush, soap, and incense for checking airflow). When they arrived at the households the workers would perform a quick diagnostic examination to determine the exact location of the problem. The workers quickly became adept at locating sources of odour, broken parts, or leaking pipes.

The majority of the complaints to the hotline were mechanical problems with the toilet, odour, flies, fans, and blockages of the urine pipes (Figure 15). Over the 16 months of problem monitoring there was an average of 66 calls per month. The most common problem during 2008 was related to mechanical failures. It was found that some parts of the turning mechanism for the toilet bowl were easily damaged from corrosion and/or inadequate

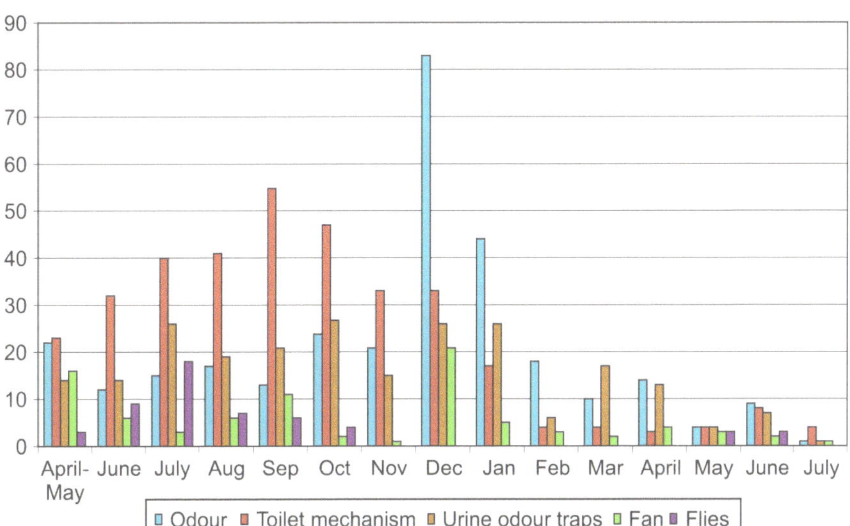


**Figure 15.** Most common problems reported to the maintenance hotline
*Source:* Data compiled from hotline database, April 2008–July 2009

strength of the materials. The springs, chains, and lever in the system often failed and had to be replaced. The SPO engaged manufacturers to provide the maintenance team with chromium-plated springs, stainless steel chains, and stronger rods so that replacement parts would be stronger and more durable. A supply of extra parts was kept at the eco-station. Sometimes the turning mechanism just needed a bit of oiling and cleaning, however more often the solution to mechanical problems was replacement of the parts.

Another common complaint was excessive odour in the toilet room or blockage of the odour-control mechanisms (odour traps and S-pipes). Reports of this problem peaked during the extremely cold winter of 2008–2009. In case of an odour complaint, the maintenance worker first needed to determine where the odour was coming from, i.e. faeces, urine, or greywater. If the odour was from faeces, the maintenance workers would check the airflow in the chute pipe by applying smoke from incense sticks and examining the chute from both the toilet and basement to make sure there was no blockage by plastic bags or other garbage. The blower fans would also be checked and the seals on the basement cabinets. Sometimes a cabinet door had been left open by accident after emptying, or a worker had forgotten to close the inspection lid on the cabinet. This would interfere with the ventilation system and could cause odours in the household.

If the odour was from urine, it could mean three things: the pipe connection under the toilet was leaking, the odour-trap was faulty, or the S-pipe in the urinal was blocked. The urine pipe connection under the toilet was a common problem that was often caused by a construction error. In many of the units, the pipe from the toilet bowl had the same diameter as the connecting pipe, making it difficult to join and seal them properly. In some cases the floor drain for the urine pipe was off centre and therefore the hose connections did not fit properly. In these cases a special, flexible hose was installed. In other cases an improved rubber seal could solve the problem.

The other major source of urine smell came from odour traps and S-pipes that were blocked by urine crystallization and the precipitation of struvite ($MgNH_3PO_4$). During operation, the maintenance workers reported that these blockages could occur as often as every month. Initially, blocked traps and S-pipes were replaced with new ones. After testing different combinations of acid and alkaline solutions, however, a cleaning solution was developed. The recommended cleaning technique was to disassemble the trap, soak it in 15 per cent hydrochloric acid (HCl) solution for 15 minutes, then brush off the struvite crystals. This work was done by the maintenance staff on a monthly basis, and required keeping extra traps in stock. An alternative household-level solution was to pour 300 mm of vinegar into each trap before going to bed, then pouring some water in the trap the next morning to flush away the loosened crystals. It was recommended that this be done every 10–15 days to prevent blockages. When visiting households for repair work, the maintenance staff would take the time to teach the users how to do preventive cleaning of the odour-locks and S-pipes using the vinegar method.

In addition to problems with struvite, the paraffin-oil odour traps required regular maintenance. After the urinal was used for a certain period, the paraffin oil became depleted, so it was necessary to add a small amount of paraffin oil periodically. The households were taught that they should add 10–15 drops of oil on a daily basis to avoid odour problems. In addition, it was recommended that the device be removed and cleaned every six months. The paraffin trap was difficult to remove and clean, however, so many households ignored this advice or called the maintenance staff to do the cleaning.

Other common problems were related to the ventilation fans in the basement and the presence of flies. The fans that were used to pump the air in the ventilation pipes could be very noisy and there were many complaints regarding the disturbance. On the other hand, there were also complaints when the fans were not working and odours started venting back into the toilet room. Flies were a problem, mainly during the summer months. Once the sealed cabinets were placed in the basement, the only way for flies to get into the system was through the toilet itself. The problem with flies was another indicator that the system was not being used properly, since flies were probably entering the system through food thrown down the chute.

When they were called in for repairs, the maintenance team took the opportunity to visit and advise the households on how to use the toilet and urinal correctly. They explained to households how to avoid future problems, particularly how to avoid odour problems by cleaning with less water and using more sawdust to keep the contents of the bin dry. The workers focused special attention on households that had strong complaints, but many times they felt that households were not listening.

## Systems level

Beyond the user interface was an entire technical system that also needed to be managed and maintained. This system included the collection pipes and bins, storage units, and the treatment plants. Operation and maintenance of this system was the responsibility of the maintenance team.

### *Routine maintenance work*

A typical day for the maintenance team consisted of inspecting faecal bin rooms, changing the bins, responding to household complaints, and reporting to the project office. Every morning, the team checked the basements in all buildings to see that everything was working properly. The bins were checked to see if they were full and that the covers were properly sealed. The fans were checked to see if they were working and that the sawdust traps under the fans were empty and tightly closed. They also checked the general cleanliness and working conditions in the basements. If there were any problems they were reported to the responsible technician and cleaned or repaired immediately by the team members.

If bins were found to be full during the morning inspection, they were emptied later the same day. In general, maintenance workers reported that they changed each bin at least once a month and sometimes as often as weekly. The higher rate was caused by too much sawdust being added by the users and also the addition of solid waste thrown into the toilet. During emptying, the bins were removed from the cabinets and wheeled to the access pit where they were hoisted out (Figure 16). The hoist was mounted on the back of a truck where a worker could stand to manoeuvre the bin into position on the

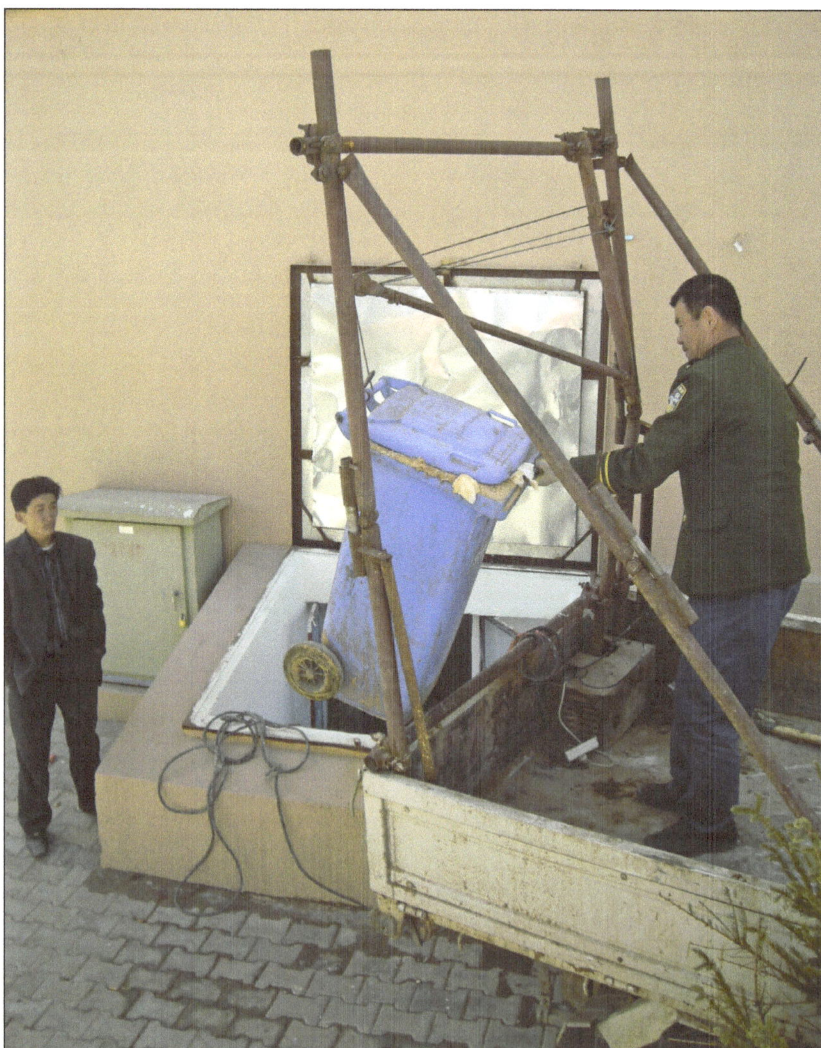

**Figure 16.** Removal of bins by using a simple hoist installed on a light truck

truck bed. The hoist system was slow and unstable, so maintenance workers were sometimes tempted to pull up the bins by hand instead. Lifting the bins approximately four metres, either by hand or with the hoist, increased the risk of spillage of faecal matter, especially when a toilet was misused and the bin was heavy with excess water. When the full bins were loaded onto the truck, the workers put empty bins in their place and double-checked that everything was properly placed. The bins were then driven to the eco-station where they were emptied at the compost plant.

The maintenance team also kept track of the urine level in the storage tanks and emptied them with the suction truck as needed, approximately every two weeks. Emptying of the tanks was designed to be once a month; however, emptying had to be done more frequently because the households poured too much water into the urinal and toilet bowl. Approximately four truckloads of urine were collected from the eco-town every two months. The eco-station was not designed with a large urine storage capacity, because the urine was supposed to be transported directly to the farmers' storage tank on the farm. Unfortunately, the farmers' tanks were limited in capacity and they could not always accept the urine. The urine was, therefore, sometimes dumped in the municipal landfill. Conversations with the maintenance workers in 2009 indicated that they had to dump the urine discretely outside the eco-town since they were not regulated to do it elsewhere. It was suggested that a larger urine tank be built at the eco-station as a buffer, however this was never realized.

**Box 3.1 Workers' voices**

In discussions with the maintenance workers in 2009, they reported that they were not very busy, but that the work was very dirty and could be physically demanding. Lifting the faeces bins was the hardest part of the job. There was a lifting machine on the truck to help get them out of the basement, but then the workers had to empty the bins themselves into the compost plant. It was very dirty and smelly work.

The workers had gloves, but that did not prevent faecal matter from getting everywhere. In summer, when it was hot, the gloves could break. One worker remembers washing his hands a lot since it was so dirty. The worker's shower at the eco-station was broken so he did not regularly wash after work. He never got sick, however, and he did not remember any of his colleagues getting sick either.

Fixing the toilets was also difficult. If the turning bowl was a problem, the entire toilet had to be lifted away to get at the mechanical parts. It could take an hour to fix a toilet, even working as a team of two. Sometimes they had to ask the households for help with moving the toilet or holding parts.

'I don't like working on the team, but it is my job and I have to do it. The project is good, except for the smell. I live here and must admit that I do not like the dry toilet. If there was no smell, then dry would have been okay.'

'The project is good, it saves water and recycles. The use of urine and compost on vegetables is better than chemical fertilizer. This project was just a test and maybe the method will be successful after several more tests.'

In addition to managing the flows of waste products from the system, the maintenance team also performed general inspection work in the apartments. Starting in the spring of 2008, the maintenance team began an inspection programme that included visiting every household every three months and detailed reporting on the overall functioning of the system. The inspection included presence of odour, whether the bowls and sawdust dispenser were working smoothly, the general condition of the urinal and odour traps, as well as checking for leakage of urine pipes. Any problems were reported and fixed.

### *Composting plant operation*

During operation of the composting plant, the maintenance team would unload the full bins from the truck and empty them into the rotating cage mixer in order to remove solid waste that had been thrown down the collection chutes. There was, however, a lot of solid waste mixed in with the faeces and workers often had to do additional sorting of the waste by using a rake. Sometimes workers had to deal with water-filled bins resulting from incorrect use of the toilets by residents who poured excessive amounts of

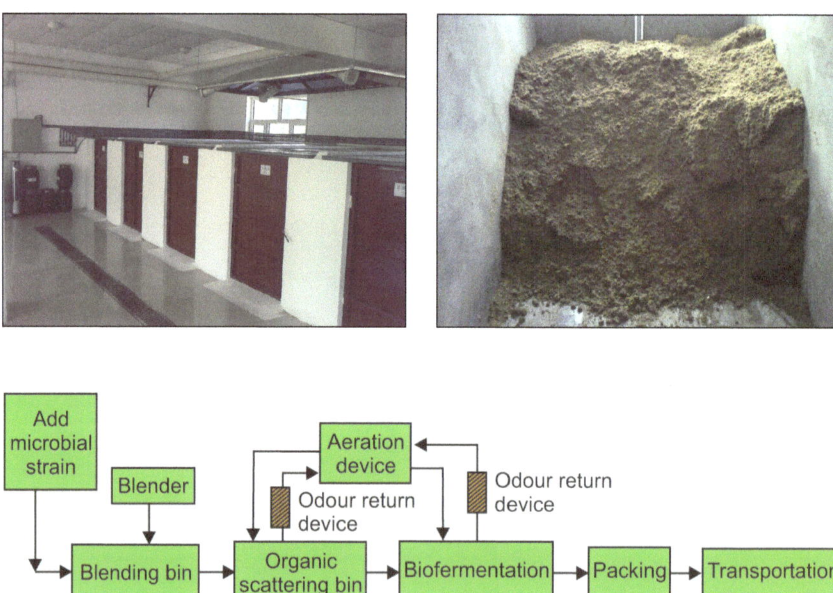


**Figure 17.** Composting plant showing the steps in the process, including material preparation, blending of the effective microorganisms, and actual fermentation, along with odour management and packing of the final product. The left-hand photo shows the 6 $m^3$ compartments, each with a red metal door with pumped aeration through small holes in the floor, containing the compost batch. The right-hand photo is a close-up of one of the compost piles in a compartment

water down the faecal chutes. The contents of these bins were poured onto a field outside the eco-station and workers disposed of any non-compostable solid waste into a garbage bin.

Once the plant was up and running, the composting procedure was adapted slightly during use so as to optimize the process. From the mixer, the sifted material was then loaded onto a wheelbarrow for transport to the composting chambers. Sawdust was added as an additional carbon source to help fuel the composting process. The aeration period was extended from four days to 25 days and the heating period adjusted to cover days 4–25 instead of only the last five days (Mertens, 2009; Mertens and Rosemarin, 2010). Transferring of the material between beds was done after 18 days instead of after just four to five days. The last ten days of the 35-day cycle were considered a resting period, allowing the compost to stabilize. The temperature in the compost was monitored twice daily and the moisture was controlled using a standard compaction method. The maintenance workers would adjust the airflow and heating as necessary to achieve the right temperatures. Weekly manual turnover of the compost materials was also used to maintain aerobic conditions. When the compost process was complete, the workers would bag the finished compost so that it could be distributed to farmers.

A study of the compost plant performance in 2009 indicated that it was possible to achieve high temperatures in the 50–60°C range for 14-day periods or longer both in the winter and in the summer months; however, the composting procedure, as practised, was not consistently able to maintain elevated temperatures. The study did show significant bacteria reduction based on total coliform bacteria as an indicator (Mertens, 2009). It was suggested that performance could have been improved by adding organic kitchen waste (the collection system was never fully developed), filling the bins completely to ensure sufficient raw material or more frequent manual aeration of the bins (ibid).

The compost plant initially suffered from odour problems when bins were delivered containing high amounts of water that had gone anaerobic. At times the smell was so strong that the staff were unwilling to work inside the plant. A ventilation system was constructed which forced the indoor air prior to evacuation through two tanks (100 l) containing HCl and NaOH solutions to absorb any ammonia or hydrogen sulphide gas. This sort of odour management is common for composting facilities located in urban areas in China.

### *Greywater treatment plant operation*

The greywater treatment plant, although built on time, was slow to come on-line. The water use by the households and thus the flow to the treatment system was much lower than expected. The underground pipes were also crushed by heavy vehicles during construction and the inspection wells were full of earth, thus blocking flow. During this period of low flow, greywater had to be bypassed directly to the pond without treatment. Yet, due to the low greywater flows and high evaporation rate in the pond, the accumulation rate in the pond was low. In July of 2007, the maximum water level had reached 0.7 m deep. It was only in August 2007 that the greywater treatment plant came on-line, once the pipes had been repaired. Only the regular treatment process was put into operation, while the reclaimed processing and chlorination step was never put into practice.

The maintenance team was in charge of servicing the connection pipes to the greywater treatment plant and an independent contractor was hired to operate the plant itself. The operator was in charge of monitoring the performance of the plant and making sure that the equipment was functional. An important function of the monitoring programme executed by the contractor was to determine the chemical and biological properties of the greywater, as well as test the operation of the treatment plant. The data produced from this monitoring programme is believed to be the first greywater data set produced in China.

The treatment plant was unable to consistently meet the Chinese greywater discharge standards which are based on concentrations of polluting substances. Testing during 2007 indicated that it generally met Total-P and $NH_3$-N requirements, but could not meet COD consistently (Zhu, 2008). A review of 2008 monitoring results for the greywater system found exceedances of COD, Total-P, TSS, and anionic surfactants at various times (Flores, 2010). Difficulty in meeting the standards can be partly explained by the exceptionally low use of water by the households and therefore low dilution of the greywater. According to an investigation of household water meters carried out between April and May 2007, the daily water use in EETP was approximately 48 l/person/day, only 60 per cent of that of the design. The Chinese discharge standards, like others around the world, are based on concentrations and not mass loadings. The fact that the plant was operating well below its design capacity probably affected the performance but this is also a comment on the inflexibility of conventional treatment systems that are usually not designed to save on water use.

In addition, performance was affected by mechanical problems at the plant which were not always taken care of promptly. The contractor did not receive much supervision and they did not carry out O&M work according to standards. In mid-2008, it was found that the secondary sediment tank needed desludging (it accumulated sludge during the 1.5 years waiting to be put into operation) and that the aeration machine in the post-treatment pond was broken. When these were dealt with, the water quality of the pond improved significantly. Aeration equipment and floating bio-baskets had been installed in the pond during the summer of 2007 as a means to reduce potential odour problems. The machines had problems with electrical failure and only worked consistently for one month.

There were also contractual problems with the operation of the greywater plant, especially during the handover period. The contractor had signed an agreement through the end of 2008 and more or less fulfilled his obligations during this period. When the handover was delayed in 2009, an oral agreement was made between the DPO and the contractor to continue operation of the plant. There is no evidence, however, that the contractor continued to work at the plant in 2009 and by mid-2009 equipment failure in the plant made it essentially inoperable. Failure to prioritize O&M is a common fate of wastewater treatment plants in developing country situations and an explanation of why sewage treatment can be so dysfunctional.

## Operating costs

The costs for operating the sanitation system at the EETP included the salaries of the maintenance workers, electrical costs for the basement fans, greywater and compost plants, purchasing sawdust, fuel for transport of reuse products, and the running of the project office. These costs were split between the SPO and the DPO, each essentially paying half of the total costs. In general, there were two main categories of costs: those for operating the treatment facilities (eco-station) and those for managing the project office.

Costs for the treatment facilities included maintenance workers, electricity, and an operator for the greywater treatment plant. The electrical costs for the ventilation fans in the basement are also included in these costs (Table 3.1). The operating costs shown are largely based on costs from 2008–2009, since the eco-station only became fully operational during this time, with the greywater treatment plant on-line in late 2007 and the compost plant in late 2008. At the height of operations, there were eight workers and their supervisor. The workers received a monthly salary between 2,500–3,000 RMB ($365–$440). Labour costs represented a substantial percentage of the total operating costs. An independent operator was also contracted to manage the greywater treatment plant.

**Table 3.1** Average monthly operating costs for the EETP system

| *Expenses* | *Cost (RMB)* |
|---|---|
| **Eco-station** | |
| Greywater plant management | 3,500 |
| Greywater and composting plant operation (electricity) | 5,199 |
| Basement fans (electricity) | 4,637 |
| Vehicles (fuel) | 4,473 |
| Maintenance workers | 21,145 |
| **SPO Office** | |
| Office staff (three staff members and an accountant) | 24,750 |
| Staff support costs (travel, phones, etc) | 2,050 |
| Office supply and utilities | 2,567 |
| **Total** | 68,321 |

(1 RMB = $0.15 as at January 2012)
*Source:* SEI budget and SPO bills 2008–2009

The remaining operating costs can be correlated with electrical and fuel consumption for both the greywater treatment and compost plants. It is difficult to determine the exact operating costs for either the greywater or compost plants independently because the electrical meters were not separated. Therefore, it is only possible to measure the total energy consumption for the eco-station. Average monthly electrical costs were 5,199 RMB ($780)/month which is equivalent to approximately 12,500 kWh (based on 0.415 RMB($0.06)/kWh). The operational costs of the basement fans were slightly less than that of the eco-station: 4,637 RMB ($700)/month and 11,200 kWh. An additional operating cost was the fuel for the vehicles for transporting the excreta from the apartments to the eco-station. Monthly fuel costs were similar to that of the basements' electrical costs.

In addition to the operating costs of the eco-station, there were significant management costs. The project office was financed by both the DPO and SPO and was run by three full-time staff, plus assisted by various DPO staff. The average monthly cost of running the project office was about 30,000 RMB ($4,500).

A team from the Environmental Science and Engineering Department at Tsinghua University was commissioned by SEI to perform a comparative economic analysis of the EETP dry system against a conventional waterborne sewage system (Zhou *et al.*, 2007, see Annex 2). Zhou performed three types of economic analyses: (1) a comparison of the construction and O&M costs of the EETP dry system (actual project) versus the equivalent costs of a conventional centralized waterborne system; (2) a comparison of the estimated construction and O&M costs of an EETP-type dry system versus the equivalent costs of a conventional waterborne system; and (3) a comparison of the cost-effectiveness of the two systems based on a cost-benefit analysis.

According to the results, the unit capital cost of the dry system was more than twice that of the centralized waterborne system: $480 versus $217 per capita. Capital cost comprised pilot tests and experiments, engineering, environmental assessment, design and construction management, civil works and equipment, and land-use fees. The difference in capital cost is mainly driven by the high cost of construction of the basement to house the dry system faecal collection system; it represents 40 per cent of the total dry system cost. The cost of the small greywater treatment plant and the composting plant also contributes significantly, resulting in unit treatment costs six times greater than that of the larger conventional centralized system.

Similarly, the study found that the O&M cost of the dry system was greater than the centralized waterborne system, by about three and a half times: $106 versus $31 per household per year (Flores, 2010). The annual O&M costs, taking into account resource recovery, came to $87 for the dry system and $18 for the conventional system using fertilizer prices from Liu (2007) and reclaimed water pricing from Zhou *et al.* (2007). The average annual per capita disposable income of urban residents in the Erdos Municipality as of 2006 was 14,000 RMB ($2,100) (Flores, 2010). If full cost-recovery was to be achieved, on average the residents would have been expected to pay 2.7–3.2 per cent of their income towards the dry sanitation system O&M. In contrast, the conventional system would have cost 0.55–0.94 per cent. With the District water rates at 3.3 RMB ($0.50)/$m^3$, the estimated annual water fees per household for the EETP and conventional systems are, respectively, $29 and $49. Together, the sanitation and water supply charges would equal 3.6–4.1 per cent for EETP and 2.1–2.4 per cent for the conventional system. According to the World Bank (2007), 'the general range of what is considered "affordable" for water services is three to five per cent of household income', therefore both systems fall within the 'affordable' range.

In the cost-benefit analysis (Annex 2) the net present value[1] (NPV) of the dry system was positive while that of the waterborne system was negative. This preference for the dry system was based on an analysis that included the following benefits for the EETP: (1) avoidance of user charges for sewage collection and treatment; (2) sales of reclaimed water, compost, and urine; (3) avoided cost of constructing wastewater collection and water supply facilities based on water savings; (4) economic benefits from water savings; (5) increased value of agricultural products based on the use of organic fertilizers. Note that the sludge from the waterborne system sewage treatment plant (STP) was not considered marketable as the STP receives a large proportion of industrial wastewater, which results in the sludge being classified as hazardous waste. The results here seem to indicate that the dry system will only be economically advantageous if there is a profit from the reuse products.

## Environmental impacts

A Life Cycle Assessment (LCA) of the EETP was performed comparing it to a traditional wastewater treatment plant (Flores, 2010). The following are the major environmental costs of the dry system.

*Use of natural resources.* Except for water, the dry sanitation system consumes greater amounts of natural resources than does the conventional waterborne sanitation system. This is in large part due to the conventional system's centralized and larger-scale design, allowing it to benefit from economies of scale in both construction and operation. In addition, the current design of the faecal collection system for the dry system is quite material-intensive because of the basements required for faecal collection and storage. The dry system transport requirements are also quite energy-intensive as the receiving farms are 40 km away from the EETP; transport of large volumes of urine/water is particularly energy-intensive.

*Discharges.* The effluent from both the dry and the conventional systems are discharged similarly, i.e. via surface soil discharge, and thus neither has direct wastewater discharges into surface water bodies. The total Eutrophication Potential of the conventional system is 3.5 times greater than that of the dry system, in large part due to the latter's recovery of nutrients for agricultural application (note that this assumes that the urine and compost are fully recovered). The dry system total Freshwater Aquatic Ecotoxicity Potential (persistent compounds if discharged into aquatic systems) is approximately twice that of the conventional system, resulting from the use of larger amounts of PVC for the separate collection of waste streams. The total Global Warming Potential (GWP) of the dry system is three times greater than that of the conventional one, resulting from the much greater electricity and diesel consumption of the dry system during operations. Additionally, the greater requirements for cement, concrete, and PVC for the construction of the dry system contribute to its greater GWP. Odour is a common complaint for users of the dry toilet, resulting from ammonia emissions from urine and likely sulphide and organic emissions from the faecal chutes. As noted above, the ventilation system of the EETP still required improvement. Both the composting station at the EETP and the conventional STP suffer from odours that can be problematic for residents in close proximity.

Any hazardous substances found in urine, faeces, and greywater are equally likely to end up in land for both the dry and conventional systems since both the liquid and solid portions of wastewater are discharged to land. Accordingly, the two systems have similar Terrestrial Ecotoxicity Potential (TEP) associated with their operations. Since construction TEP contributes only a small percentage, the total TEPs are similar for the two systems.

*Resources recovered.* The dry system has superior resource recovery capabilities in the case of nutrients and organic matter. Both systems are, however, capable of recovering water for irrigation and other purposes. The EETP greywater system is expected to be capable of producing higher-quality reclaimed water as it does not receive urban stormwater and the associated high contaminant loads; on the other hand, because of the low dilution rates, the greywater tends to be more concentrated. The collection system of the Dongsheng conventional STP, while designed to receive only wastewater and not stormwater, is more susceptible to illegal/unplanned discharges, and is thus more likely to have lower-quality effluent.

## Health risks

Operation of the EETP dry system posed several health risks for users and workers from exposure to faecal matter. Key exposure points occurred during toilet use, handling of faecal bins, on site composting, urine collection and transport, and application of reuse products to agriculture. During toilet use, two potential sources of health hazards were the faeces and sawdust. Particularly for users who found the use of the toilet challenging (children, women, and the elderly), misuse of the UDD toilet may have led to faecal contamination outside of the turning bowl. In addition, since cleaning the

UDD toilet required minimal use of water, it may not have been sufficiently cleaned or disinfected to minimize exposure of users to residual faeces.

The trapping of sawdust and faeces in the turning bowl may have been problematic in that the mixture could serve as a breeding ground for pathogenic organisms. A study by Williams *et al.* (2008) on the persistence of *E. coli* in butcher shop floors found that damp sawdust in contact with *E. coli* increased the survival rates of the bacteria. This is consistent with the findings from a study done by the Environment Science and Engineering Department of the Beijing Aviation and Astronautics University, commissioned in this project which concluded that the sawdust serves as a good medium for cultivating microorganisms (Zhu, 2008). Sawdust was a concern particularly for women with regard to exposure of the genital area during toilet use. Fine sawdust was reported to be re-suspended which could then adhere to the exposed skin. One possible health impact of such an exposure is skin infection, however there was no documented evidence of this and it was not clear how much of a health risk this truly represented. Sterilization treatment of the sawdust with ozone prior to distribution was recommended to reduce health risks. Sawdust was sifted and air dried prior to packaging in this project.

One particular area of significant public health risk for the EETP dry system was the handling of faecal matter by the maintenance personnel. At each step in the faecal collection and composting procedure, the workers were exposed to raw faecal matter, and there was ample opportunity to contaminate surfaces and tools. Furthermore, incorrect use of the bins by residents who poured excessive amounts of water down the faecal chutes resulted in heavy water-filled bins that required special handling. To minimize risk from handling the faecal materials and compost, workers were provided with protective clothing, which included rubber boots, work jackets, work pants, gloves, caps, and dust masks (Mertens, 2009). Tools dedicated to the composting plant were also provided, as well as washing facilities for the equipment and the workers. The compost plant workers were trained on proper hygiene practices (e.g. no smoking and frequent handwashing), which required strong reinforcement.

The public health risks from the use of composted faeces for agriculture can be minimized through proper operation of the composting process, appropriate application techniques by farmers, and the practice of hygienic food handling by consumers. In the case of urine and greywater, the potential for health risk was primarily attributable to faecal cross-contamination. Some users found the separation of faecal and urine streams difficult, making cross-contamination a potential problem. Excessive use of water to clean the toilet bowls could also have resulted in faecal-contaminated wash-water being directed into the urine tanks. Finally, pipeline misconnections, both intentional and otherwise, made cross-contamination of both urine and greywater systems a reality at the EETP. Even before the switch to flush toilets, some families installed their own flush toilets, which were connected either to the urine or greywater pipelines.

The more complex piping system of source-separation systems required more careful installation than a conventional mixed wastewater system and this level of care and inspection was lacking in the EETP. An investigation in April 2008 revealed that the plumbing in the EETP was often done in a haphazard manner, increasing the risk for cross-contamination from cross-connections and blockages (Selke, 2008). Construction quality control, strict enforcement of the dry sanitation system design (e.g. making pipeline cross-connections illegal or in violation of the building contract), and additional education of the households are some of the measures that could have been used to reduce the risk from cross-contamination.

CHAPTER 4

# Research and development

Since this project was a R&D pilot project, there were some limitations with the initial design and several parts of the system required upgrading and retrofitting. As mentioned in Chapter 3, the majority of the problems were related to the toilet riser and odour from the collection system, therefore most of the upgrading work went into fixing these problems.

The project was a source of much learning both in the development and testing of prototypes and in full-scale implementation and maintenance. In particular, the urine-diverting toilet underwent modifications from a turning bowl to sliding plate system over the chute opening and the urine-odour lock was modified from an oil-seal lock with standing urine to various plastic sheath design air locks with no standing urine. Ventilation of the faeces bins also underwent development including the original sponge-lined bin cover to the sealed cabinet system and improved basement pipe and fan alignments venting to the roof level. Many corrections were added when it was discovered that the original installations were faulty and had not followed the blueprint designs. Considerable experience was gained in the area of indoor air pressure management since toilet ventilation was directly affected by kitchen and bathroom fans and opening of windows as well as outdoor air pressure changes caused by gusting high winds and low external air temperatures (down to –30°C). Frozen ventilation, water, and urine pipes were also experienced, mainly because of inadequate thermal insulation. Critical data has been derived regarding ventilation pipe diameters for roof exhaust depending on volume of air-flow and pipe stack height.

The original first four buildings had faeces bin ventilation riser pipes that were 75 mm in diameter which proved to be inadequate to vent the upper two floors under conditions of air pressure shifts. The rest of the buildings were equipped with 110 mm diameter riser pipes. Toilets were originally equipped with low-cost metal fittings which rusted and wore out prematurely, although the original design called for stainless steel springs, chains, and metal parts.

Additional research was also conducted on the reuse potential from the waste products collected at the EETP. There were a number of large-scale agriculture field trials using faeces and urine fertilizer, and the results were disseminated through training sessions and workshops with local farmers. Although reuse of waste products never reached the levels that were envisioned at the beginning of the project, the data generated provide a solid basis for future work.

## Toilet model improvements

The original toilet model installed at the EETP had several flaws, specifically relating to the turning-bowl mechanism, cleaning of the bowl, and the use of sawdust. Firstly, many of the bowls did not consistently turn 180 degrees so that faecal matter would be deposited on the sides of the bowl. This problem was often related to poor installation of the toilet or mechanical failure of the parts due to corrosion. Aside from problems with the mechanical parts, many users found that the toilet was difficult to operate. The turning bowl and flushing knobs were difficult to use, especially for children and the elderly. They often did not weigh enough for the toilet ring to force the lever mechanism to turn the bowl or have enough strength to pull the sawdust-flushing lever.

From a maintenance perspective, cleaning the bowl was problematic since in order to reach the bowl one hand was needed to press down on the toilet seat, leaving only one hand free to clean the bowl. The bowl also proved difficult to clean as faeces stuck to the bowl and dried in place. Secondly, the use of sawdust also proved problematic since it was difficult to dispense and could be re-suspended and escape from the toilet bowl. As noted earlier, users were also concerned about the health consequences of sawdust. In order to solve some of these problems, the toilet was adapted and retrofitted twice. Finally, in 2009 a new toilet, a modified Separett model, was introduced with a significantly different design.

### *Second toilet model*

In order to fix the problems with the turning bowl, both the Dongsheng Project Office and the building company requested that a new toilet model be developed. This second model used the same porcelain toilet but with a few adaptations. The first change was that the turning mechanism for the bowl was connected to the lid instead of the seat ring. A connecting rod linked the lid of the toilet to the turning bowl so that when the lid opened it pulled the bowl over. When the user finished and put the lid back down, the lever system turned the bowl back. In this model the bowl could be cleaned simply by opening the lid and the weight of the user on the seat was no longer a problem. Another improvement in the second model was the use of a rotating wheel to dispense sawdust instead of the gated box and push button. A turn of the crank dispensed a consistent amount of sawdust into the bowl without requiring much effort on the part of the user.

This prototype was tested and improved several times before the final version was finished in June 2006. Two of these models were then installed in households for trial, and performance was reported as satisfactory, especially for the sawdust dispenser. There were still some mechanical problems, however, regarding the turning-bowl mechanism. The torque on the plastic lid was quite high and there were worries that eventually the mechanism would fail or break the lid. Due to these concerns, a third prototype was proposed for further retrofitting.

### *Third toilet model*

The third toilet model sought to correct problems with the turning mechanism and concerns about the sawdust dispensing system. This model was based on the same porcelain model as its predecessors. Due to the frequency of complaints regarding the turning bowl and related difficulties in cleaning, it was decided to remove the bowl completely. Instead, a movable plate was introduced to cover the faecal hole and chute when the toilet was not in use. Similar to the second toilet design, the lid was used as the lever for moving the plate. When the lid was opened the plate slid back from the opening to allow for defecation, and when it closed the plate slid back sealing the chute (Figure 18). The prototype was completed in mid-2007 and tested in 22 households, where it received positive evaluations.

This model also meant that the addition of sawdust by the user was no longer necessary, or even desirable. Removal of the turning bowl changed the airflow velocity in the chute so the down-draught was not enough to overcome the up-draught from the chimney effect. This meant that re-suspension of sawdust added by the users became a problem. To overcome this, sawdust was added directly to the bins by the maintenance team. In this way, the suspension of fine sawdust particles in the shaft was minimized and the user environment was kept cleaner.

The third prototype had several advantages in that it was mechanically simpler than the turning bowl design, required fewer material parts for the toilet, and rendered the addition of sawdust by the user unnecessary. The maintenance workers were also happy with it since it required far less servicing. In some cases it also improved the odour problems of the toilet since the lid sealed tighter. For example, one fourth floor apartment reported a completely improved odour situation after receiving the new toilet model. Most of the mechanisms for moving the plate and lid were plastic and there

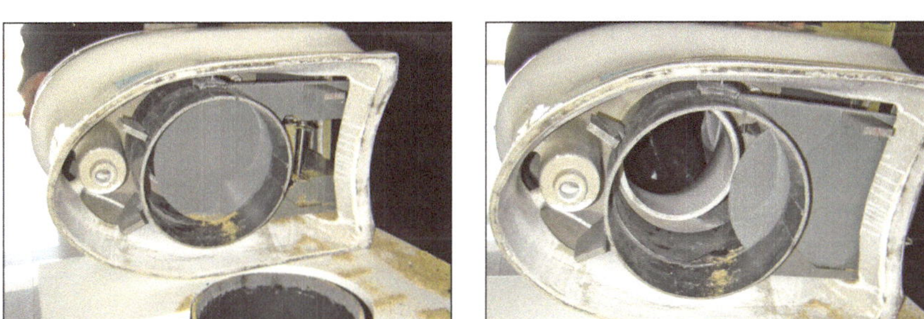

**Figure 18.** Cross-sections of the third toilet model, showing the sliding plate design

were concerns about durability and the quality of the material. Further prototypes and testing were therefore recommended before a complete retrofit of all apartments could be undertaken.

### *Separett toilet model*

During 2008, retrofitting efforts focused on understanding and improving the ventilation system as a key step in improving user satisfaction and eliminating odours. After continued user complaints, however, it was decided that a commercially available dry toilet should also be tested. The Swedish company Separett has been manufacturing UDDTs for over 30 years and is one of the world's leading manufacturers of urine-separating toilets. In early 2009, the company donated five demonstration toilets for modification and installation in the EETP. The original Separett model used is a free-standing toilet where the faeces are collected in a container within the toilet and manually removed when the container becomes full. For the EETP installations, the bottom of the collection container was removed so that the faeces could fall into the drop chute (Figure 19). The bottomless container (a plastic pail) was easily removed for cleaning. Similar to the third EETP model, the Separett model used a sliding plate to cover the opening to the collection container when not in use. By sitting down on the seat ring the sliding plate would open. The urine outlet from the toilet was easily connected to the existing urine system in the EETP buildings. Of particular importance from the user perspective was that the toilet had its own two-speed evacuation fan that created an airlock over the faecal chute and urine opening, thus blocking odours from entering the toilet room.

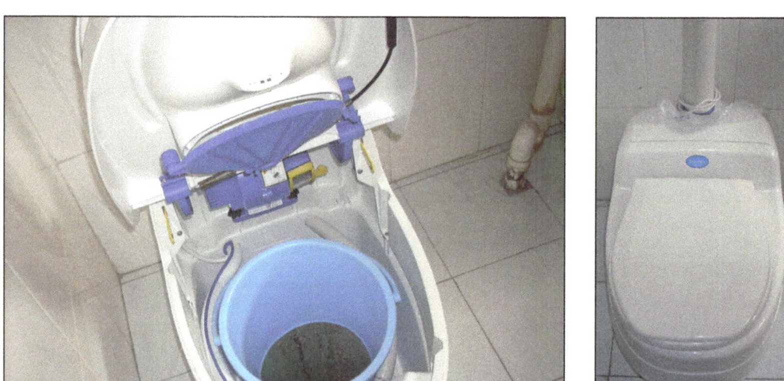

**Figure 19.** The Separett model, with bottom removed, connected to the drop chute, and the removable bottomless pail to ease cleaning. These toilets continued to be used in one stairwell and four floors following the project in 2010.
*Source:* SEI

The Separett model was installed in one stairwell with four households, during a three-month trial period. When the residents were interviewed at the end of this period, they were quite satisfied with the functioning of the toilet. It was agreed to extend the trial period for an additional year into 2010.

## Ventilation retrofitting

One of the major reasons for odour problems in the apartments was the poorly functioning ventilation system. The ventilation pipes were supposed to draw the air out of the toilet rooms, down the chutes and vent it to the roof. It was difficult, however, to achieve the required airflow rates in the vent pipes and maintain the downward airflow in the chutes. The use of kitchen fans, changes in outside air temperature, or windy days could affect the air pressure enough that the ventilation system periodically failed to function as designed. In an attempt to overcome these problems, the design was modified and retrofitted a few times.

In the original design, the ventilation pipes were connected to the lid of the collection bins. A branch pipe from each of the four bins connected to the horizontal trunk pipe (Figure 9). In this design, the axial fan was located at the end of the trunk pipe, making the junction to the vertical ventilation pipe. The airflow in this design was lower than expected, due to resistance in the system. In order to reduce this resistance, a second arrangement was tried in which the branch pipes were connected directly to the chute instead to the bins; however, subsequent use showed that this design also had shortcomings. Since the branch pipe was directly connected to the faecal chute, materials such as sawdust, toilet paper, and garbage thrown down the toilet would get sucked into the pipe and block it.

The opportunity for a new ventilation system arrangement presented itself when it was found that the faecal collection bins were also not functioning properly. After one year of operation, the foam seals on the bins had deteriorated and the steel mechanisms for the lids had rusted. The damage to the foam sealing meant that air was leaking into the basement, interfering with the proper flow of ventilation and causing odour problems in the basement. To fix the problem it was decided to replace the movable bin covers and place the bins in sealed cabinets (Figure 20). The cabinets were made of polymer-coated aluminium plate with wood or steel framing. The cabinet doors and pipe connections were sealed with airtight rubber. In order to avoid opening the doors frequently, an observation hole was provided on the top of each cabinet. During the beginning of 2007 all of the movable bin covers were replaced by cabinets. Although the costs and space requirements for the cabinets was greater than the bin covers, they significantly improved the air quality in the basements. Tests conducted by ventilation consultants showed that replacement of the bin covers with cabinets reduced the ammonia levels in the room by nearly half (Zhu, 2007). The cabinets also greatly reduced the

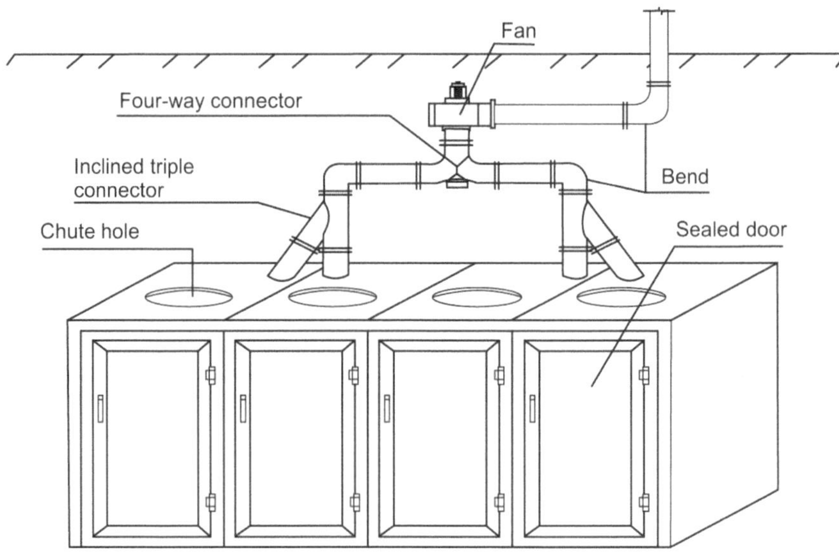


**Figure 20.** Third type of vent-pipe arrangement with sealed cabinets housing the faecal bins

number of flies in the bins and made it easier to control them if they became a problem.

Installation of the cabinets allowed for a third arrangement of the ventilation pipes to be installed. In order to achieve a more uniform distribution of airflow, the new arrangement shifted the location of the fan to the middle of the trunk pipe and reconfigured the pipes so that the fan was pulling an equal distance from each of the cabinets (Figure 20). This design also remedied the clogging problem of the second design by reconnecting the branch pipes to the sealed containers.

In connection with the installation of the cabinets, a series of ventilation studies were performed on the system. The aim was to identify problem areas and potentials for further retrofitting if needed. Most of the results showed that the actual flow rate in the system was lower than designed. Part of this was under performance of the fans, but the studies also discovered that many of the ventilation pipes higher up in the buildings had been poorly installed, causing restrictions in the outgoing airflow. For example, in buildings No. 1 to No. 4, the main ventilation pipes were installed with a 75 mm diameter pipe instead of 100 mm called for in the design. This caused resistance in the shaft to be four times higher, and corresponding airflow lower. Additional inspection found misaligned fans and pipelines, pipes with multiple bends, and other construction-related problems that caused high resistance in the system. In particular, the use of flexible branch hoses to connect the bins to the trunk pipelines led to reduced airflow. This problem was partly remedied with the third piping arrangement and the installation of stronger centrifugal pumps in some of the buildings. In many buildings, however, the poor construction of the system meant that each toilet room would have to be retrofitted individually, making a complete retrofit costly.

## Reuse

The goal of the ecological sanitation project was to establish a system of reuse and recycling for the waste products from the eco-town. The project never reached its goals of full-scale recycling, however it did provide valuable research experience on the fertilizing potential in the excreta, logistical aspects of such a system, and local perspectives influencing reuse practice. This section describes the results of the field research, the implementation and reuse practices achieved during operation of the dry toilet system, and finally personal reflections on the reuse system by residents and workers in the eco-town.

### *Field trials*

A number of large-scale field trials using human excreta from the EETP were conducted by the Erdos Soil and Fertilizer Station (ESFS) and the Dongsheng Agriculture Technology Extension Service Centre (ATESC). The objectives of the trials were to measure the nutrient value of the compost and urine produced at EETP, test methodologies for their use in agriculture, and demonstrate reuse to local farmers. The tests performed in 2007 indicated that the urine solution and the compost mixture generally met standards for agricultural applications, even though their nutrient content was lower than expected due to excessive amounts of water and sawdust. Later testing of the compost produced by the eco-station onsite composting system (completed in late 2008) showed that the compost had lower N, P, and K content than chemical fertilizer on a mass basis, but was comparable to composted garden waste (Mertens, 2009).

Field trials were conducted using corn and potato during 2006 and 2007 (Liu, 2007; Liu and Zhao, 2007). Application of both faecal compost and urine was tested in increasing doses (from zero to 12,000 kg/hectare) on a number of test plots. The results from the test plots were compared against conventionally fertilized and unfertilized crops. The results of these tests were generally promising. Corn fertilizer with only urine produced 11–25 per cent more yield than unfertilized crops. If only composted faeces were applied, the yield was 23–40 per cent higher than unfertilized corn. A combination of both urine and compost resulted in yields similar to that of traditional fertilizer crops (e.g. manure and chemical fertilizer). The results from the potato experiments were similarly positive.

## Reuse in practice

As part of the research programme, ATESC conducted a series of demonstration and training courses explaining the benefit of using sanitized human urine and faeces as fertilizer. Between the winter of 2005 and spring of 2006, fifteen training courses were held in which about 300 local farmers participated. In addition, the maintenance team of EETP was trained and encouraged to use the demonstration gardens near the eco-station. The maintenance workers grew a variety of vegetables for their families in these gardens and used urine and compost as fertilizer.

Large-scale reuse of urine was not achieved during this project. The use of urine as a landscaping fertilizer was forbidden by the local housing association and there was no apparent demand from local agriculture. Therefore, it was taken by the maintenance team to the municipal landfill.

Reuse of faeces from EETP was more successful than urine, although the system did not reach the potential envisioned at the beginning of the project. Prior to the compost plant coming on-line at the end of 2008, the faecal matter was composted outdoors on a farm 30 km from EETP and eventually incorporated into the fields. Due to the distance to the farm, however, some of the faeces were also dumped at the municipal landfill. After the compost plant became operational, bags of the finished compost were given to several local organic farmers for use in their greenhouses. Since the compost did not meet Chinese standards for organic fertilizers, the EETP was unable to sell it, but as a free product the farmers willingly used it to cultivate a variety of vegetables. The farmers reported being satisfied with the EETP compost, although SPO staff had doubts about whether they would purchase it on a routine basis. The compost quality would probably have been improved if organic kitchen waste had been included in the process, but the green-bag programme only got started in 2009 as the push to replace the dry toilets reached its height.

## Perspectives on reuse

In general, it can be argued that there was not enough public awareness and promotion of the reuse aspects of the eco-town project. The majority of the residents were not interested in agriculture or the environmental benefits of their toilet. A survey of residents in 2009 showed that they had little interest in the agricultural reuse aspects of the EETP dry system. Only one respondent selected 'produces organic fertilizer' as a benefit of the dry system and 74 per cent had never visited the eco-station (Flores, 2010). Only 40 per cent admitted to knowing that their excreta were used in agriculture. Maintenance workers felt that the households were more interested in solving the problems with the toilets at the household level and did not care so much about reuse. In addition, government officials did not prioritize reuse aspects or promote legislation to enable reuse. In fact, the government restricted the use of urine fertilizer in public places for fear that it would create odour problems.

Perceptions regarding the agricultural acceptability of human fertilizers remained mixed, although a majority of residents did not think it was acceptable to use human excreta on agriculture. Only 20 per cent found agricultural application of urine acceptable, and 40 per cent in the case of faeces (Figure 21). This may be a reflection of a subconscious acceptance, rather than a conscious and public one, of human excreta application to agriculture, or perhaps it is a reflection of changing attitudes as people move up the economic ladder in China. There was also concern about using treated greywater to irrigate the gardens around the EETP; 45 per cent of residents were against this practice, mostly due to fear that it would smell.

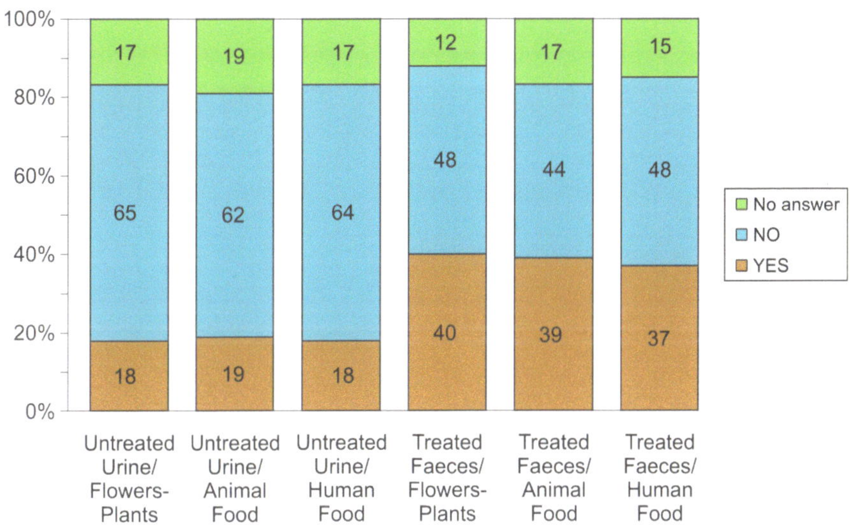


**Figure 21.** Survey results of user acceptability of applying untreated urine or treated faeces on various types of crops. This is in response to the question: 'Would you purchase/consume the following items if urine/faeces is applied [as listed in the figure]?'
*Source:* Flores, 2010

# CHAPTER 5
# Social acceptance

The apartments in the EETP were sold by the developer on the open market starting at the end of 2004. Advertisements for the area highlighted the green environment and recycling eco-system (Figure 22). The advertising campaign introduced the eco-toilet to the buyers as the 'advanced Swedish technique'. The apartments sold quickly as they were priced below the average retail value for downtown Dongsheng. The new owners were required to sign an agreement to use the dry toilet. Based on the advertising leaflets and discussion with residents afterwards, it seems clear that few households actually understood the nature of the dry toilet. Prior to their purchase, the majority of the new owners were not aware of the fact that the EETP was a R&D project, or that effort would also be required from the users to ensure a successful operation of the toilet.

Given their low level of prior knowledge, the residents of the EETP were patient and supportive during the first years of the project. The initial support stemmed from the residents' belief that the dry toilet was an ideal toilet for the eco-town. According to a resident spokesman in 2009, they had shown their support during the initial years by constantly raising suggestions for improvement. Support dwindled, however, as problems with the system persisted and solutions were slow in coming. This chapter presents the users' experience with the system and how changing opinion would eventually lead to a switch to a flush toilet system.

## Living with dry toilets

Before getting into a discussion about user acceptance of the dry toilet it is necessary to understand a little about who the residents were and where they were coming from. Although originally envisioned as housing for resettlement of displaced farmers, the majority of EETP residents were middle class or the parents of middle class children. The majority also had private flush toilets before they moved to the EETP. This change in target users was partly due to the economic boom in the Dongsheng area as a result of coal mining. The area has experienced unprecedented urban growth in the last ten years. When the project started in 2003, the GDP of the Erdos municipality was 4.9 billion RMB ($735 million) and average income per capita of the urban residents was 6,900 RMB ($1,035) (Government of Dongsheng District, Erdos Municipality, 2003). In 2007, however, the municipal government reported that GDP had reached 115 billion RMB ($17 billion) and per capita income of urban residents had increased to 16,226 RMB ($2,400). This level of GDP

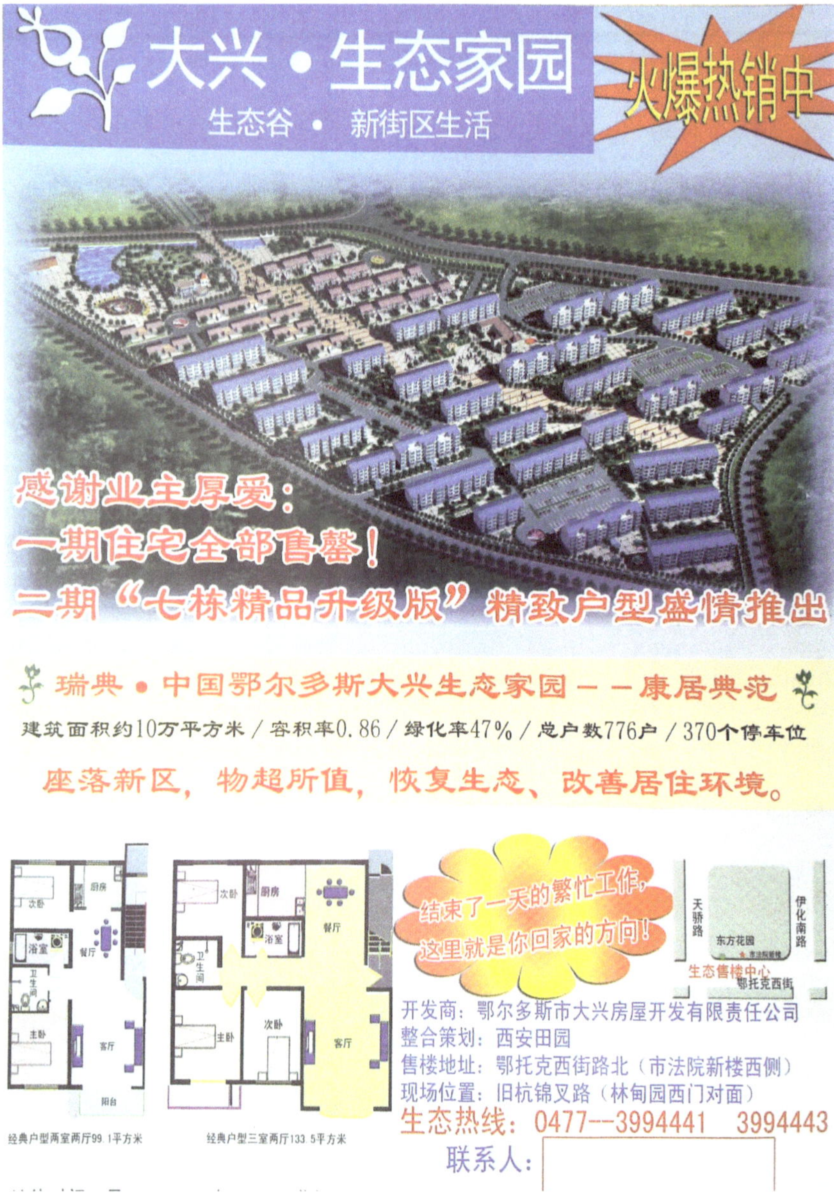


**Figure 22.** Advertising leaflet to market the apartments in the Erdos eco-town stating, 'Typical well-off living with 47 per cent green area, located at the new city area. Value exceeds the cost. Recover ecosystem and improved resident environment'
*Source:* Daxing Estate Development Co.

put the city in the same league as Beijing and the National Bureau of Statistics ranked Erdos 28th among the most economically powerful cities of China (Ordos On-line, 2010).

The rapidly changing social and economic situation in Erdos resulted in corresponding changes in living standards and aspirations. The population of Erdos now dreams of a modern city with all the associated benefits that urbanization can bring. The urban residents in the Dongsheng District associated dry toilets with a lower standard of living and the old city that they were trying to leave behind. Flush toilets represent the modern standard, as indicated by the fact that waterborne systems were installed in all new multi-storey housing built in the city between 2007 and 2009. The local government appeared to agree with this view of flush toilets as the improved and modern alternative since all new public toilet facilities installed in 2007 in the downtown Dongsheng District had also been equipped with water-flush toilets.

Another result of the economic growth in Dongsheng was public investment in infrastructure such as water supply. In 2006, a water supply pipeline from the Yellow River was opened, providing much more water to the Erdos residents. The frequency of water rationing and cuts to the water supply decreased significantly afterwards. Although improvements in water supply probably reduced the perceived need for dry toilets, residents said that they often stored water in their bathtubs for toilet-flushing and other purposes in case the water supply was temporarily cut off. Interviews with residents in 2009 indicated that they did not see water shortage as a significant problem.

Besides water savings, another driver for the EETP had been agricultural reuse of waste products. Economic growth and the shift in target populations also undermined the significance of this argument for dry toilets, however, at least from the user perspective. As shown in Chapter 4, the new middle class residents of the EETP showed little interest in the agricultural reuse aspects of the dry system. Lacking drivers such as perceived benefits of water savings or agricultural reuse, the primary driver of user acceptance was based on their day-to-day interaction with the toilets and urinals in their homes.

Users' experience with their dry toilets was not always positive. As was shown in Chapter 3, there were regular complaints about odour and mechanical problems with the toilets. A report from the social worker at the end of 2007 stated that only 13 per cent of residents were satisfied with the system. Further studies after the 2008 retrofitting work found high dissatisfaction with the toilets and urinals (Flores, 2010). Only eight per cent of survey respondents indicated that they would recommend the dry system and the vast majority would prefer to have a flush toilet installed in their household. Households generally felt ashamed of their dry toilets and thought that it was negatively affecting the value of their apartment (Figure 23). There were even some residents who preferred to use the nearby public toilets rather than their own.

A number of different surveys showed that residents found odour to be the most serious problem with the toilet. The results of a questionnaire to households in January 2007 found that 67 per cent of respondents had an odour problem and 14 per cent thought it was serious. In a survey by Flores in 2009, bad odour (48 per cent) was reported more than twice as often as other problems, such as inconvenience of use (18 per cent) and difficulty in cleaning (11 per cent). In general, the odour problem was reported to be worse during bad weather, windy days, or extreme heat. A significant social consequence of the odour problem was that the friends and relatives of residences did not want to visit. This was a source of stress and embarrassment in many families. There were even reports that some people became sick because of this stress. Eventually, this would be one of the driving arguments that the users would use to change the system.

It must be noted, however, that the dry toilets were not the only problems that residents for the EETP were experiencing. An independent evaluation of the project in 2008 by the University of Science and Technology in Beijing (USTB) discovered a long list of faulty items in the original building construction. These included varying pipe diameter, construction and quality not following the original blueprints, inadequate and faulty electrical installations, lack of drainage around the buildings causing waterlogging in basements, inadequate insulation of water and drainage pipes resulting in freezing, and blocked greywater drainage pipes due to soil accumulation in the brick inspection wells. The design of the system could not take into account the unanticipated occurrence of such poor workmanship and lack of building inspection. Poor

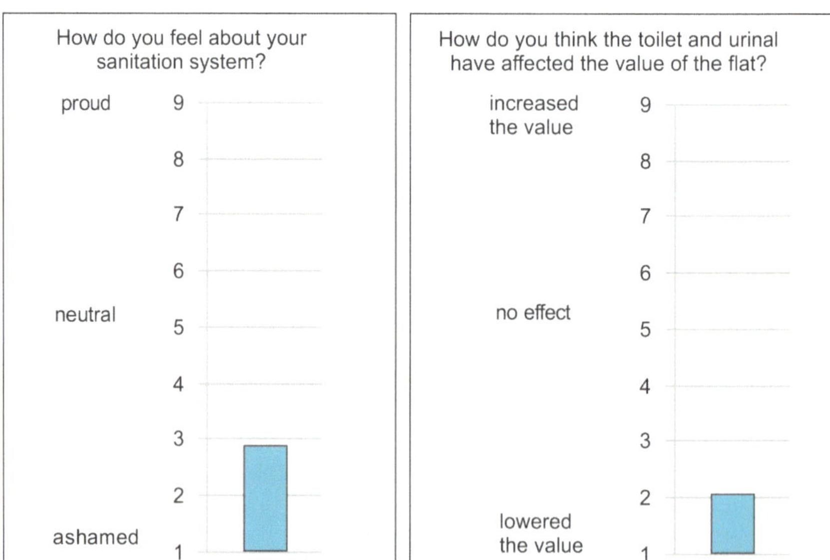


**Figure 23.** Results from the Spring 2009 survey regarding user perceptions of the dry sanitation system. Left side: average user feelings about the dry system. Right side: average perception of the effect of the dry system on the value of the apartment.
*Source:* Flores, 2010

**Box 5.1 Residents' voices**

***Man around 35 yrs***

I moved into the eco-town because of the dry toilet system and gas heating. I had heard of ecosan before and appreciate that the eco-town concept is based on recycling. I am happy with the dry system and do not think that it smells very much, although I know that it is worse on the fourth floor. The toilet can be troublesome and the urine pipe can get blocked and smell bad. However, it does save water!

***Woman around 35 yrs***

I saw the advertising for the eco-town and was convinced to move in. I did not understand the concept of a dry toilet before I purchased the apartment. I did not receive training on the toilet, only a poster with pictures explaining how to use it. The toilet is smelly and the turning bowl does not work very well. The dry toilet is inconvenient and difficult to clean. I do not like to clean the toilet because the dry faeces and sawdust get stuck in the chute and I have to scrub to get it clean. It also caused problems with visitors since it is embarrassing to explain how to use the toilet.

***Man around 35 yrs***

I live on the second floor and moved in during 2005. These toilets have many flaws. First, they are not suitable for children under 10 years of age. Second, the smell is just horrible. Third, they are inconvenient to operate, very often I have to get my hands dirty and push down the faeces through the pipe. Fourth, it is not very nice to invite guests because the whole apartment smells bad and then it is not easy to explain for guests how to operate it. Fifth, the maintenance of the toilet is bad and when *emptying,* the faeces get splattered all over the walls on the inside of the toilet. Finally, flies flourish in the apartment and it is not very pleasant. I would prefer a flush toilet.

***Woman 40+ yrs***

I have lived in my apartment on the third floor since August 2006. I am afraid that the sanitary situation might endanger my health. It is a terrible place to live and it gets worse when it is windy or is raining outside. On some occasions when the electricity is not working, the fan in the basement stops and the bad smell gets even worse. The bowl system inside the toilet does not work very well. When *emptying,* the faeces splatter all around the walls of the underlying pipe. The faeces and the moist sawdust get stuck and build up and this makes the free area through the pipe smaller and smaller. Sometimes I must use my hands to push down the faeces and that is not exactly high-tech. The urine gets stuck on the inside of the pipes and it crystallizes and creates blockages and a terrible smell. With the kitchen fan on, the smell gets even worse. Big flies flourish in the apartment. It is impossible to invite guests.

***Man 50+ yrs***

I moved into this apartment on the first floor in the winter of 2006. The whole eco-sanitation project is unreasonable in its design and operation. It is a desk-product with good intentions but it has three big flaws. First is the bad smell. Second, it lacks any economic benefits since the local government has to pay for sawdust, electricity for the fans, and collection and transport of the faeces and urine to the landfill. Third, it is not very convenient for senior citizens.

*Source:* Report from Swedish Embassy visit 10 June 2009 and personal interviews September 2009

construction quality led to cracks in apartment walls, settling sideways, leaking drainage pipes, and accelerating wear and tear on the buildings.

## Road to flush toilets with onsite treatment

Discontent with the dry toilets led some families to remove their dry toilet and install a flush toilet without approval. These flush toilets were connected to the greywater system or urine pipes. In 2006 there were four such toilets in EETP, and by the end of 2007, 15 families had changed to water-flushed toilets without consulting with EETP management. According to the social worker, one of the main reasons for the increasing change was that there was no penalty for change or enforcement rules regarding keeping the dry system. Some people changed and told their neighbours how good their flush toilet was, and when the neighbours saw that the government did nothing, they also changed. The social worker warned the SPO that if nothing was done there would continue to be more flush toilets.

There were two causes to the discontent surrounding the dry toilet. The first was that there had not been enough user training and awareness-raising about the value of the system and how to use it properly. Despite the efforts of the social worker, the SEI annual report in 2006 noted that insufficient effort had been put into promotion of household acceptance. The second was the continuing technical problems related to the toilet and ventilation system. Although the retrofitting study in 2008 achieved some further improvements in odour control in two test buildings, the majority of their findings suggested that improvements could only be made by replacing toilets and fixing piping problems on an individual apartment basis. The report of this study stressed that a root cause of the problem was that the system required properly functioning infrastructure and exposed the inadequacies caused by the poor original construction and inadequate inspection. The solution was not a quick fix, but would involve a prolonged period of retrofitting and replacement in all apartments.

The retrofit work during 2008 also discovered a growing resistance and lack of patience on the part of the residents. The study team reported that it was obvious that residents were tired of expert visitors who just talked without explaining or improving anything. Very few households expressed interest in the retrofitting work and some even ignored the communication about not using the toilets during the retrofitting work in the basement.

In late 2008, frustration led to the residents forming a household committee. The mandate for the committee was to assist households with the relationship to the service companies responsible for eco-town management, e.g. providing security, cleaning, garden services, and maintenance. Their responsibilities were to employ a company as caretaker of the sub-division and supervise their daily work. In addition, the committee was supposed to defend the legal rights of the households.

The committee inherited a difficult situation with high user dissatisfaction and an ongoing boycott of the standard service fee for apartment living. All residents are supposed to pay this fee for the maintenance of the housing area. The fee is calculated based on services rendered and generally includes building maintenance and solid-waste collection. Many households at the EETP did not want to pay the fee because they were not satisfied with the dry toilet and the maintenance company. As part of their management responsibility, the household committee tried to persuade the households to pay the fee (which is paid directly to the service companies), but they also decided to take action to improve the situation in order to avoid further boycotts.

As soon as the committee was organized they started gathering information on household opinions. Although there were a number of good things about the sub-division, such as the abundance of green space, bright apartments, and parking for cars, the committee also found many complaints. The negative aspects of the eco-town were the poor quality of the buildings and the dry toilet. Users understood that the dry toilet saved water, but they were also concerned about having to pay for the electricity it used and the maintenance fees for the workers to service the toilets. Besides being inconvenient to use, residents also felt that the odour from the dry toilet was unhealthy and the sawdust had bacteria which could make people sick.

Due to the strong household complaints against the dry toilet, the committee started to take action. They talked to the SPO and the DPO. They had a meeting at the SPO and raised some of their concerns about the disadvantages of the dry toilet, especially regarding costs, odour, ventilation, and responsibility for long-term operation. Most importantly, the members expressed the emotional stress and troubles they felt were caused by the dry system and demanded compensation. They also approached the Dongsheng government to raise the same concerns.

Pressure from increasingly impatient residents corresponded with the handover deadline for the project in 2009. Questions regarding the costs of retrofitting and related management responsibilities certainly played a role in the decisions taken in 2009. At the end of 2009, SEI was to transfer full responsibility for the project to the Dongsheng government. As this date approached, the government began to express doubts about the maturity of UDDT systems for multi-storey buildings. In a meeting with the SPO in May 2009, government officials expressed their preference for a flush system and suggested that they were only willing to continue the dry system if Sweden would pay for toilet replacement and the maintenance fees. Since project funding for the EETP had already been extended for an additional year, the Swedish partners were not willing to agree to these terms.

In June 2009, the Dongsheng District Government agreed to the households' demand for flush toilets and began replacing the UDD toilets and urinals. This was done in response to the mounting pressure from the households, despite the ongoing improvements to the system and the offer of various dry toilet alternatives to the current UDD toilets and urinals. The new system is a

DEWATS which retains the onsite decentralized nature of the project using the small-bore pipes from the apartment buildings and an onsite water treatment plant plus compost plant for sludge and kitchen wastes. By October 2009, all the dry toilets at EETP had been removed and replaced by low-flush toilets (4–4.5 litres per flush). The government also funded the construction of an on site treatment plant with both anaerobic and aerobic steps using effective microorganisms with a capacity of 500 $m^3$/day.

The Separett toilets (described in Chapter 4) installed in the flats in one stairwell continued to function well with good user acceptance for over two years before they were replaced with flush toilets in 2011.

CHAPTER 6

# Lessons learned

The mother to success in research is discovery and innovation. Quite often research breakthroughs occur by chance and due to errors or mistakes, and it is the observant and creative scientist that gains from these experiences. In fact, Nobel Prizes are often the result of following up on such discoveries that are rooted in 'failed' experiments. When it comes to infrastructure and engineering projects, the situation is usually the complete opposite. When a project fails to turn out as planned, most proponents and financiers will tend to quit sooner or later and choose to take a low profile. As a result, little publication, discussion, or social and technical learning occurs from the experience. It is exactly this sort of discussion that is lacking within the water and sanitation sector that is so riddled with mishaps and dysfunctional systems. Engineers Without Borders publish annually their *Failure Report – Learning From Mistakes* (EWB, 2010). This is the first step to social learning, an element that has been generally lacking within the sanitation sector. Indeed three recent books highlight just how riddled with failures the sanitation sector has been (Black and Fawcett, 2008; Benidickson, 2007; George, 2008).

The taboo aspect surrounding sanitation has made it a difficult subject to become a household topic discussed by policy-makers, constituents, and consumers. Without the dialogue, little innovation and development will occur and we can even get to the point that a fatality rate of 5,000 children per day due to inadequate water and sanitation becomes a taboo subject (Rosemarin, 2007).

It is therefore of importance to emphasize that this book is a story about the need to innovate within the sector of urban sanitation and it describes the details surrounding the challenges, both technical and social, that were experienced. The following is an attempt to analyse the lessons learned and to provide recommendations to those that will venture down this path again in the future.

Essentially, there are four areas or clusters of factors that can impact on such projects. These are institutional arrangements, technology development, social issues/stakeholders, and external factors. Figure 24 shows how these sets of factors sequenced in time during this project. Reality often dictates that these four groups of factors cannot be properly integrated from the start in order to minimize risks of failure, and this results in increased vulnerability for the project, especially if it is attempting to be innovative and depends on changes and new developments in technology, capacities, people's attitudes, and policies.

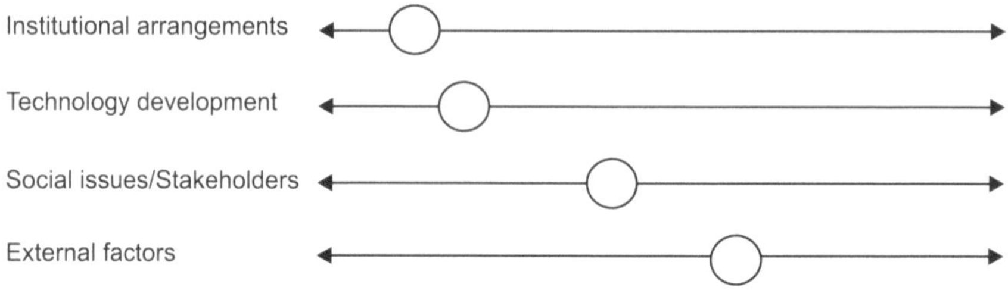


**Figure 24.** Timeline of significant factors during the project. The circle represents when the activity or factor began to be significant in the project

## Institutional arrangements

Ownership of the project was shared by the building company, Daxing Estate Development Co. and the Dongsheng District Government. This rendered the project vulnerable since it became obvious towards the end that neither were interested in taking over the project in the long term. Attempts to set up a holding company that would maintain O&M based on a fee schedule were not successful due to the relatively high expenses.

There was an inadequate process surrounding the need to make space and time for testing and R&D in order to ensure that the project could succeed. A demonstration phase was planned but the building company was more interested in finishing off the buildings to get them sold as soon as possible. This might have been better regulated through a legal agreement.

The management structure of the project could have been stronger on several fronts. Decision making, leadership, management, and project ownership on the Chinese side was inadequate, and the communication structure within the project was somewhat inflexible because of the top-down structure from the Chinese side. The agreements/contracts between the building company and Dongsheng Government – especially regarding quality control of installations – was inadequate. The power relationships had several negative effects on project management and transparency and there was a lack of supervision in the construction work. The buildings were constructed all too quickly with many different work teams involved in the installation of ecosan equipment and the plumbing and electrical installations. To alleviate quality control problems there should have been a permanent chief technical advisor onsite with the power to stop construction until corrections could be carried out. The project did have senior supervisors but these were not empowered with the capability to stop construction.

There may have been advantages if the Swedish partner had entered the project via the national government as opposed to entering at the local level. This could have ensured that the objectives of the project were implemented throughout by both the local government and building company. The nature of the project being essentially one of R&D was weakened by the fact that there was no Chinese lead research institution (although several were involved). The strength of the public–private partnership which was created in this project was not sufficiently nurtured by either of the Chinese lead partners in order to help achieve the objectives of the project.

## Technology development

The multi-storey urine-diverting dry sanitation technology chosen for this project required a high level of craftsmanship, which was lacking. In general, the entire building project – including all installations – was characterized by unacceptably poor construction quality and there was a glaring lack of building inspection. Since the technology had not been tested at this scale before there was a need for a demonstration phase under real building conditions. This was not made possible by the way the project was set up with the building company. As a result, the project could not benefit from a proper set of feasibility studies. The technology of multi-storey, ventilated dry toilets was (and remains to this day) still immature, although it has been successfully developed elsewhere at a smaller scale in several projects. There was a need for more training of the construction workers, plumbers, and users. Odour became a serious issue for the households and eventually became a project-killing factor. For such a project to succeed, one must have the user-interface right so that users will have a positive experience with the system – this was not the case.

For this project to succeed, the toilet design and associated ventilation needed to be sufficiently robust to allow for both incorrect installation and use. That is, the unit itself needed to be able to remove odours even if construction was faulty and even if the user did not follow instructions. The solution was discovered towards the end of the project in using the Separett toilet that has a self-contained ventilation capacity.

The dry toilet used in this project was inconvenient for the users, especially when it came to cleaning of the toilet and application of sawdust during each defecation. The technology problems could have been solved if there was a little more time for the project and if the building company was interested in repairing faulty installations.

## Social issues and stakeholders

The question of who pays for O&M versus who benefits from these services requires a strong connection and sense of ownership, which was lacking in this project. The government was not willing to reduce water fees for the households in this project so that they would be able to afford to pay O&M fees. The households felt the potential economic burden in taking over the project, while at the same time not seeing any benefit compared to the alternative of flush toilets. There were no incentives provided by the local government for saving water or reuse of the products from the system. To succeed, the project needed champions among the households and increased participation and education. The users should have been better educated to support the dry toilet concept and understand/appreciate the reasons for why it was being developed in this arid part of China. There was a general lack of desire among households to use eco-sanitation in a modern apartment. The negative attitude against the use of the UDD toilet was not directly proportional to the odour problems. The two investigations in January and April 2007 showed that only about half of the toilets had odour problems. There was a general bias among households that flush toilets were superior, based on convenience and aesthetics.

## External factors

The foundation of the project at the start was lack of water supply for a major urban area. Access to water then increased during the project, at least temporarily, thus removing the project's original *raison d'être*. The multiple changes in governing mayors in Dongsheng reduced the political support that was generated at the start. The project was originally to be a large-scale implementation of dry toilet technology in simpler buildings but the project changed to multi-storey buildings due to the unforeseen rapid urban development in the Erdos area. The boundary conditions of the project were in flux and became less favourable over time while the project was unfolding, with the changes in water supply, changes within the target group, and the weakened Chinese partner interest. The attitude of the target stakeholder group shifted during the project due to rapid urbanization, market shifts, and a drastic increase in the standard of living.

## Tipping points

There were several key events or tipping points that contributed to the failure of this project as follows.

*Water shortage no longer a problem.* Water rationing in Dongsheng was stopped during the project because increased groundwater extraction capacity was installed and the 100 km water supply pipeline to the Yellow River was completed. The most important driver for the project – water shortage – was at least temporarily removed.

*Odour problems.* Freezing of ventilation pipes occurred during the extreme winter of 2007 when all of China experienced record low temperatures. The rooftop vent pipes in this project had no thermal insulation and became blocked with freezing water-vapour crystals, causing indoor odour problems. The single most important feedback in sanitation systems determining success or failure is odour.

*Stakeholder approach not followed.* The project was organized with the local government in control and implemented by a building company. A stakeholder approach involving consumers was not possible since the apartments were to be sold on the open market. This, in general, is the demise of urban environmental projects, since stakeholders are not normally involved from the start. Not having the 'buy in' from the tenants meant risking the project if things were to become challenging.

*Founding of the household committee.* As the project progressed, the households created a committee in order to represent themselves. Although common elsewhere in China, this was something the local government was not really prepared for. Exactly how democratic this committee was and what methods it used in order to produce change are not really important. The fact is the committee provided an ultimatum to the mayor when the project was coming to an end and dictated they would not be willing to take on any added costs for retrofitting, operations, or maintenance.

*The standard of living increased in Erdos.* Enormous and rapid changes in the standard of living occurred during the project with the increased revenues from coal mining. Dongsheng and Erdos shifted from being a poor, dark, and dingy urban area to an expansive bustling city with a building boom like that of Shanghai and Beijing. The GDP of Erdos in 2010 was the second highest in China after Shanghai. This changed the attitudes of the households such that dry toilets were thought of as something backward.

## Killing factors

Several key factors that contributed to the failure of the project, so-called 'killing factors', are worth explaining.

*Inadequate design preparation and implementation.* The most significant factor in determining the fate of this project was immature design of the ecosan and toilet system and its sensitivity to poor construction quality which was also exacerbated by the lack of building inspection. In general, the entire housing complex suffered from lack of skilled labour and the rush to build during the urban building boom in this city. One factor that should not be underestimated is the inability to build in this part of China during the cold winter period. This shortens the length of the year for implementation by about 25 per cent. The building phase of the project was carried out too quickly and there was no time to carry out the proper testing in order to create good workmanship routines and to fully test the sanitation system, especially during a cold winter, before further implementation.

*Inadequate institutional arrangements.* The project was not set up to empower the government and SEI with sufficient control. Communication channels between the partners were insufficient to achieve the objectives of the project. Too much responsibility was given to the District Governor and insufficient power and responsibilities given to the project managers. When complaints were made regarding construction errors, there was a general disinterest on the part of the building company, Daxing Estate Development Co., to take responsibility for the poor workmanship and to agree to repair the incorrectly installed facilities. This may have been due to the lack of competition in Erdos and the relationship the company had with the local government. The local government failed to apply sufficient pressure on the building company to correct critical faults in plumbing and ventilation piping, key sources of odour. There was also a lack of interest on the part of the local government to take over the project or even to try to organize a holding company that would take over the O&M following the exit by SEI.

*Failing to convince the households.* Odour detected by the households is probably the most important factor that can make or break an urban sanitation project. The ventilation system for the toilets was sensitive to air pressure changes within and outside the buildings. Any sub-standard installations were therefore vulnerable to recurring odour problems.

Within the households, there was a lack of pride in maintaining their toilets and residents saw them as an embarrassment when they had visitors who had to be instructed on how to use them. The residents were thus unwilling to take on the costs for O&M and the local government was not willing to provide a tax break for the residents for not being connected to the municipal sewage system. There also developed a decrease in the level of confidence among households since the retrofitting improvements took too long.

The households did not clearly understand that the project was a full-scale R&D activity and when they began to realize this they lost patience and withdrew support.

Regarding dissemination of information, the real estate company provided inadequate information to potential buyers, so people bought apartments under false expectations, with no knowledge about the sanitation system.

## Lessons learned and ways forward

What then could have been done differently in order to increase the chances of a long-term success of this experimental project? And what then would be the recommendations from this project to others in China and elsewhere in the world interested in installing alternative sanitation systems in urban areas?

The comments and recommendations can be summarized into five areas:

- targeting the users;
- project ownership and leadership;

- planning and learning processes involving stakeholders and local institutions;
- design and craftsmanship in plumbing and building installations;
- dedicated O&M.

*The targeted users.* The experience from the Erdos Eco-Town Project provides a clear picture as to what the major challenges can be in providing alternative sanitation services to apartment dwellers in order to save on water and reduce environmental impact. To request urban residents to change their personal attitudes and toilet habits requires much more effort than asking them to sort and recycle solid waste. Sanitation has more to do with people's personal behaviour and the challenge is that people, especially urbanites, tend to avoid any discussion on this subject. This remains a central stumbling block in the process of introducing innovative change within this sector. As a result, the sector remains conservative and slow to respond to the need for change. This project was not designed around a set clientele of users since the residents appeared on the scene as market buyers. The building company and real estate agents did not want to take on the complicated process of describing the dry toilet system to potential buyers. A weakness was therefore built in from the start in that the users were not dedicated to the project.

*Project ownership.* In an ideal world, when it comes to project ownership and leadership, a project of this kind requires a dedicated and stable 'home' unaffected by changes in local politics. When it comes to institutions in urban settings that are set up for this sort of challenge, these can take several forms. A central characteristic needs to be the element of ownership by the residents themselves or an association representing them. Without this sense of ownership, residents will tend to lose interest in the challenges at hand. Indeed the success and failure of similar projects in Sweden has hinged on the element of ownership. The residents can, for example, take on a central role in planning and execution of the project, making demands on the architect and builder. They can then set up a holding company or buy the services of an O&M facility, or even be responsible for O&M of their own toilet and urinal systems.

When the residents in the Erdos project became organized, the municipal government was not prepared to accommodate this new element of governance. No solution relating to ownership was properly discussed so that the three parties (government, residents and building company) failed to see how improvements could be made and the responsibility shared. The government failed to live up to its original commitment to lead a project that would save water and reduce environmental impacts. The building company failed to deliver on dedicated and long-lasting collaboration. The residents were left with the responsibility but without the institutional tools to succeed. The only thing that they could do was to deliver an ultimatum to the local government that they were unwilling to take on the costs themselves of the present sanitation system and they demanded a waterborne system.

The solution the mayor then took was to invest in a waterborne adaptation of the present system using the already-installed small-bore pipes and onsite treatment. This was, in itself, a sort of new statement of ownership by the government, out of necessity to solve the stalemate and to achieve a long-term result. This decision was good in that it reinforced the original commitment by the government to support a sustainable alternative to save water and protect the environment while listening carefully to the stakeholders. So, in a way, the project took a new turn in a positive direction. Whether this new system will lead to others following this example remains to be seen, but it has certain advantages over conventional systems since large sewer pipes and pumps are not used and the decentralized nature can lead to optimization of overall treatment capacity and even reuse.

*Planning the project.* Part and parcel of the ownership aspect is the planning component and the process of choosing the sanitation system that the users want to have installed and are willing to work with. This requires a dialogue and is an important step in the overall learning process by examining alternatives. Most urban centres around the world are not set up for this sort of planning dialogue and 'standard' solutions are decided on by architects and engineers. The users pay for these without questioning them or finding out if there are, in fact, alternatives. Private homeowners are in a better position to plan alternative systems to both save money and protect the environment. Still, it is a challenge to find out just what the alternatives can be and only recently a proper compendium on technologies was published (Tilley *et al.*, 2008) along with an assessment of health aspects (Stenström *et al.*, 2011). Methods for sustainable sanitation planning although well developed for rural settlements have not been as developed for urban centres and have only recently been described (Lüthi *et al.*, 2010).

The project was shifted by the mayor of Dongsheng from single and double storey courtyard housing for displaced farmers to market-based multi-storey apartment buildings for urban dwellers and a decision had to be made as to whether the project should go full-scale or be restricted to a demonstration for testing. The debate centred around whether a smaller-scale test demonstration project could produce the necessary learning required by the EcoSanRes Programme. The advantages of learning from a full-scale application were several, even if the risks were higher, so the decision to go ahead with a full-implementation project was taken. Although the project planned for a demonstration phase for testing, this was not given priority by the building company. So, if there was one built-in weakness, it was this one. To avoid this, a contract demanding a period of initial testing and development would have been necessary in such a project and this should have been insisted upon by the local government.

The project probably could have benefited from greater involvement of the central government in China. This would have placed the project at a higher level of governance and such aspects of testing and development might have been given a higher priority. A mechanism for the management of the project could then have been worked out with the oversight of, for example, the Ministry of Urban and Rural Construction and the Environmental Protection Agency. This would have changed the attitudes and dedication of the project partners at the local level.

*Design and craftsmanship.* It was stated above that toilet systems need to be robust and designed to provide a minimum standard of service, even if they have been installed or used improperly. The technology requirements for dry toilets in multi-storey buildings are very different from the standard waterborne toilet systems. When it comes to odour management, the flush toilet has a water lock, thus preventing much of the odour from the pipes below to enter the air space in the bathroom. When it comes to building norms such as pipe diameters and ventilation systems, such do not yet exist for multi-storey dry toilet systems. So for dry toilets to compete with flush toilets, the toilet itself needs to be able to manage odour in order to convince the user. This can be done, for example, by using a small self-enclosed evacuation air fan placed in the toilet that ensures that the air space around the user and in the bathroom itself has no odour. This combined with urine diversion can ensure an odour-free delivery system. The system with centralized fans used in the present project was sensitive to incorrect pipe installations but also to changes in air pressure both within and outside the buildings. Of utmost importance in such a project is the level of craftsmanship in the installations, the ability to follow blueprints, and the respected role of building inspection. In the case of the EETP, there was no owner that could insist that incorrect and sloppy installations be redone by the building company.

*Operations and maintenance.* Of course for any sanitation system, large or small, O&M are the key to long-term successful use. If this is not properly organized in an urban apartment complex, the system will sooner or later fail. The ability to organize and pay for this service returns us again to the role of strong ownership. So even if the government in Dongsheng decided to take on the next step of the project with a sort of DEWATS, a formula for O&M would still be necessary for long-term success. This also includes the financing of this activity.

*Sustainable sanitation.* Although this book may leave the reader with the conclusion that waterborne sewage is the only practical solution for cities, and that people's behaviour surrounding sanitation facilities and their unwillingness to try new approaches demands that waterborne systems continue to be chosen, there are alternatives to today's conventional systems that are being tested. The approach to sanitation up to now has been generally to find affordable ways to dispose of sanitation wastes. This is not a sustainable approach, knowing that population densities and contamination risks are high, but also that the products of sanitation (both water and nutrients) are in fact valuable for society in urban agriculture and should not be thought of as waste. A wealth of literature based on first-hand experience is being produced by SuSanA on the sub-sectors involved. Decentralized waterborne systems with gravity-fed small-bore pipes, septic tanks with biogas, and fertilizer production from the sludge and wetlands to absorb the final effluents are ways of avoiding costly conventional less sustainable systems. The separation of storm water from black and greywater provides a basis for reducing the volumes that need to be treated for pathogens. Wet composting of slurried sludge can produce sufficient thermal conditions to ensure pathogen kill-off, and this is necessary for both animal manure and human manure prior to their safe reuse in agriculture. Pathogen-free manure and sludge are all too uncommon today.

When it comes to areas that are periodically flooded or that have serious droughts, approaches to water supply and sanitation need to be rethought if the solutions are to be more sustainable. Sanitation systems designed around safe and environment-friendly reuse will look different from those designed around disposal. Much of the urban world still does not have networked sewage systems and use onsite flush systems with septic tanks and pit latrines that need to be maintained and emptied. The options for upgrading these systems to optimize performance and even provide safe reuse remains one of the most challenging areas in human development today.

As the world's urban population continues to increase, especially in the developing countries, there is much to be done to make sanitation more sustainable, at the same time continuing to satisfy the needs of the urban dweller. It is our hope that this book has in some way provided further insights into the overall process of social learning towards these goals.

# Annex 1
# Job descriptions of the project experts

*Ecotoilet and Ventilation Expert*

- reports to the Project Manager;
- develops methods and technologies for the management of excreta of humans and animals (collection, storage, primary treatment);
- adapts ecosan technologies to specific conditions in existing buildings (retrofitting methods);
- carries out in-service training of project staff;
- manages ecosan installation during the implementation phase.

*Solid Waste and Eco-station Expert*

- reports to the Project Manager;
- develops methods and technologies for the management of solid waste (sorting at source, collection and storage);
- develops and tests the concept of 'neighbourhood eco-station';
- develops methods for safe storage of materials in the eco-station;
- develops compost and secondary treatment of excrement of human, animal and organic wastes from households (warm compost and vermiculture systems);
- performs environmental impact assessment of the eco-station (air and water).

*Agriculture Reuse Expert*

- reports to the Project Manager;
- collaborates with local farmers;
- develops methods and technology for agricultural reuse of organic and products from the eco-station;
- performs studies on soil quality and commercial crops.

*Greywater Expert*

- reports to the Project Manager;
- works on the efficient use of the water supply system;
- develops greywater treatment alternatives;
- provides special consideration for winter conditions (freezing of surface soil to 1.5–2 m depth);
- designs the drainage system;
- provides for recycling and groundwater recharge of treated greywater;
- designs a storage system for the treated greywater.

*Physical Infrastructure Expert*

- reports to the Project Manager;
- performs detailed town planning;
- works on the architectural design of the buildings;
- designs the water supply system;
- designs the drainage system;
- designs the roads and plans the earth and landscaping work.

*Temporary R&D Staff – International and Chinese*

- report to the SEI Project Supervisor;
- perform R&D collaboration with experts team;
- carry out specialized training of local project teams;
- test and demonstrate various project components;
- report on progress;
- participate in international liaison.

# Annex 2
# Cost-benefit analysis of the EETP ecological sanitation system[1]

## Introduction

Since the 20th century, the water flush toilet has been used across the world, and wastewater treatment technology has become more and more advanced. The rapid growth of population and cities has created increased water pollution, however, and something like 90 per cent of the sewage in the world is discharged into the environment without significant treatment. One billion people use water flush toilets, but 70 per cent of the black water is inadequately treated (Chinese Environment Protection Agency, 2005).

In China, every year the amount of sewage created in towns and cities reaches nearly 30 billion tons which represents over half of the total amount of wastewater produced. About half of the sewage generated in China is treated in China and the rest is discharged directly into rivers and lakes (Helmer and Hespanhol, 1997).

Conventional sanitation and drainage systems dominate, but these have met obstacles and problems in their practical application. This is mainly because of the following:

- The cost of construction and O&M of the waterborne system and its sewers and sewage treatment plants is expensive.
- An average of 15,000 litres of clean water is needed to flush human excreta per person per year, which means a significant water loss which in some parts of the world contributes to water scarcity.
- In the conventional sanitation system, human excreta are diluted using clean water and then discharged into sewers, which results in the discharge of the nutrients from human excreta as a pollution source.
- As scientists discuss strategies to solve the global water crisis, they consider existing problems in the current conventional system again and question the sustainability of the system. Many countries are now trying to apply ecosan systems and reconstruction of conventional drainage systems (Winblad and Simpson-Hébert, 2004).

An ecosan system is an alternative to the conventional system, where the focus is on containment, treatment, water conservation, and recovery of nutrients from the human excreta. The features of ecosan systems are as follows:

- Human excreta and other organic waste are treated by natural or low-energy approaches, for instance, composting.
- The nutrient materials, i.e. nitrogen and phosphorus, are recovered safely and become a part of a closed nutrient cycle.
- Ecosan systems have a lower water consumption than conventional ones, and the wastewater produced from the system is treated and reused, for instance in irrigation, recreational ponds, etc.

As a part of the EcoSanRes Programme, a combined body including local government, SEI and Daxing Estate Development Co. constructed an ecosan system in the Haozhaokui (HZK) community of Dongsheng District, the China–Sweden Erdos Eco-Town Project (EETP) from 2003. Residents began to move into the community by 2005. The HZK community was the largest urban ecosan system of its kind in the world. The project consisted of 43 buildings with four or five storeys and equipped with UDDTs in every apartment. The number of households totalled 832 and the population was 2,912. The technical essentials and assumptions for the CBA are described as follows:

- Dry toilet system in that faeces and urine are collected and stored through different pipes and storage devices are applied. No black water is produced in the system.
- Faeces are composted with organic waste from the community, and the fertilizer is used for agriculture. The collected urine is also used for agriculture after appropriate storage and dilution.
- The greywater from the apartment is collected through a small-bore drainage system and treated in the community decentralized wastewater treatment plant. This consists of secondary treatment including a primary settling tank, a bio-film reactor, and final settling pond, and the effluent is designed to meet the national discharge standards. Part of the effluent is treated through additional treatment, i.e. a filter process, and the reclaimed water used for land irrigation and recreational ponds in the community.

The application of ecosan in an urban setting, especially involving source-separation systems is a novelty for China, so the aspects of available techniques, user acceptance, benefits, costs and future application potential need to be studied. These systems affect not only pollution control, but also real estate investments, environmental impacts and benefits, and economic impacts, all which can influence policy-making, and technology application for environment improvements in local areas.

A cost-benefit analysis and comparison between the EETP ecosan system and a conventional sanitation system was carried out. The results are therefore relevant for projects with a similar scale.

## Methodology

### *Method of economic evaluation in the study*

Human activities, including policy-making and project development, have influence on the environment and natural resources. An economic evaluation tries to assess the technical and institutional feasibility of a project, relative to some other alternative. Several evaluation technologies are often used, including cost-benefit analysis (CBA), cost-effectiveness analysis (CEA), cost-utility analysis (CUA) and cost minimization analysis (CM). In this study, CBA is applied considering resource scarcity, pollution control, environmental improvement, and the project's contribution to the country's welfare.

In the CBA application, the environmental impact of the project is also considered. Most countries and international organizations employ CBA in project analyses (Belli *et al.*, 2001; Zhou, 2001). CBA is based on the country and societal considerations, which are different from project financial analyses that only include the private sector or group benefits in market prices and economic costs. Because of market distortions created by either the government or the private sector, transfer payments must be removed in CBA. Meanwhile, the project's externalities are identified and quantified in money units where possible and included in the economic analysis as project costs or benefits.

## Criteria used in CBA

The economic net present value (ENPV) is the basic economic criterion used in CBA. This forms the basis for whether we accept or reject a project, and reflects the net contribution of a project to the country or society. The ENPV of a stream of costs and benefits is a number that results from discounting the values of the stream at a given social discount rate. It is equivalent to the number that results from the following expression (Belli *et al.*, 2001; Zhou, 2001):

$$\mathrm{ENPV} = \sum_{t=0}^{n} \frac{B_t - C_t}{(1 + i_s)^t}$$

where the social discount rate is $i_s$, the benefit in year t is $B_t$, the cost in year t is $C_t$, and $n$ is the time horizon. The ENPV of a stream is equivalent to the amount that would have to be invested today in order to obtain a return $i_s$ for $n$ years. According to the guideline, the social discount rate, $i_s$, should be less than eight per cent for environmental protection projects in China (Construction Ministry of China, 2006). In the study $i_s$ is eight per cent.

The expected ENPV of the project must not be negative when discounted at an appropriate rate. For the comparison of mutually exclusive alternatives, the project with higher or highest ENPV will be given the most acceptance (Belli, P. *et al.*, 2001; Construction Ministry of China, 2006).

## Results and discussion

### *Identifying benefits and costs of the EETP ecosan system and conventional sanitation system*

The schematic scenario and components of the EETP ecosan system and conventional sanitation system are shown in Figure A.1. The effluent quality of the two systems meet the 'Discharge standards of pollutants for municipal wastewater treatment plants' (GB 18918-2002) level one, class B (Chinese

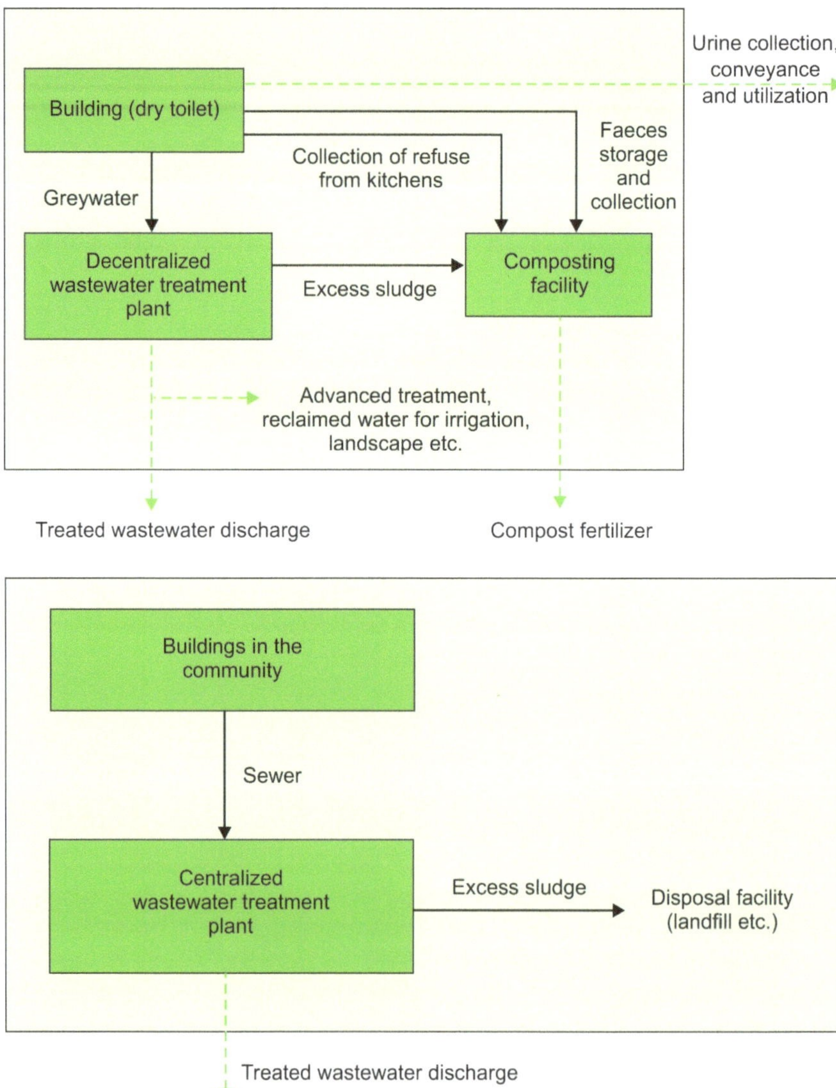


**Figure 1.** EETP ecosan and conventional sanitation systems

National Standard) (Construction Ministry of China, 2002a). The reclaimed water quality from the EETP ecosan system meets the 'Code for Design of Wastewater Reclamation and Reuse' (GB 50335-2002) (Chinese National Standard) (Construction Ministry of China, 2002b).

Based on the components of the two systems, the benefits and costs of the EETP ecosan system are summarized in Table A.1, where the calculated time horizon is 22 years, including a two-year period for construction (Zhou, 2001; Shanghai Municipal Design Institute, 2000).

Following Chinese guidelines and the local survey for Dongsheng District, water demand is assumed to be 80 l/person/day (Office of Underground Water Management in Dongsheng District, Erdos City and Office of Water Saving in Dongsheng District, 2004; Construction Ministry of China, 2002c). Due to dry toilet system application in the EETP, the actual water consumption was 47.7 l/person/day based on household surveys, the ratio of water saving being 40 per cent.

The benefits and costs for the conventional sanitation system are shown in Table A.2. The calculated time horizon and period of project construction are the same as for the ecosan system. The wastewater treatment plant (WWTP) capacity in the scenario is 40,000 $m^3$/d, which is based on the present sewer system in Dongsheng District. The calculated water consumption was 80 l/person/day. The sewage from every household discharges into the urban sewer system connected to the WWTP.

In the identification and calculation of the benefits and costs for the EETP ecosan system, some external benefits and costs are not included in the study because it is difficult for them to be quantified in money units. For instance, energy consumption will decrease in water purification, water supply, wastewater conveyance, and treatment because of water savings from the dry toilet system, which results in decreased coal consumption in the power station, lowering $SO_2$ and $CO_2$ discharges and resulting in air quality improvements. Additionally, treated wastewater that meets certain standards will improve local the water environment and promote tourism, which is difficult to quantify as well.

## Economic comparison and analysis between the EETP ecosan and conventional sanitation systems

The results of the economic criteria calculation for the EETP ecosan and conventional sanitation systems are shown in Table A.3.

When the social discount rate is eight per cent, the ENPV of the EETP ecosan system is more than zero, which means that the project is accepted or feasible. The ENPV of the conventional sanitation system, with eight per cent social discount rate, is less than zero, i.e. the conventional sanitation system is not deemed acceptable or feasible. The reasons for infeasibility include the lower wastewater tariff, higher construction costs, the lack of wastewater reuse, and the selection of social discount rate in the conventional sanitation system.

**Table A.1** The benefits and costs of the EETP ecosan system

| | **Benefit of the project** | |
|---|---|---|
| | *Item* | *Benefit per year (RMB)* |
| Direct | Cost of O&M in wastewater treatment plant (residencerate 100%) | 40,552.96 (discharged wastewater flow: 47.7 l/person/day; community population: 2,912, average wastewater tariff: 0.8 RMB/$m^3$) [i] |
| | Income from reclaimed water (residence rate 100%) | 27,145.14 (reclaimed water flow): 82.634 $m^3$/d, price of reclaimed water 1 RMB/$m^3$ [ii] |
| | Compost fertilizer and urine (residence rate 100%) | 66,000 |
| | Residual value | 392,306.75 (ratio of residual value 4%) [iii] |
| External/ indirect | Decrease cost from facility construction of wastewater and solid waste treatment | 1,828,849.08 (decrease discharged flow: 32.3 l/person/day; community population: 2,912) [iv, v, vi] |
| | Decrease cost from facility construction of water treatment | 376,320.00 (decrease discharged flow: 32.3 l/person/day; community population: 2,912) [iv] |
| | Decrease cost from garbage and excess sludge disposal (residence rate 100%) | 22,778.54 (decrease discharged flow: 32.3 l/person/day; community population: 2,912 [vi] |
| | Decrease cost from operation of wastewater treatment plant and sewer (residence rate 100%) | 33,824.11 (decrease discharged flow: 32.3 l/person/day; community population: 2,912) [ii, v] |
| | Decrease cost from operation of sewer treatment plant and water supply (residence rate 100%) | 70,941.40 (decrease discharged flow: 32.3 l/person/day; community population: 2,912) [iv, vii] |
| | Net increase benefit in local industries from water-saving (residence rate 100%) | 11,434,953.60 (90.9 RMB/$m^3$ water) [viii] |
| | Decrease value of environment deprivation from water pollution (residence rate 100%) | 400,493.18 (discharged flow: 80 l/person/day, community population: 2,912, value of environment deprivation 4.71 RMB/$m^3$ wastewater) [ix] |
| | Net increase benefit using compost fertilizer and urine (residence rate 100%) | 10,000 [x] |
| | **Cost of the project** | |
| | *Item* | *Cost per year (RMB)* |
| | Investment | 9,807,668.79 (Based on actual data. 40% of gross investment in first construction year, 60% in second year) |
| | O&M | 253,498.33 [iv, xi] |

**Table A.2** The benefits and costs of the conventional sanitation system

| | **Benefit of the project** | |
|---|---|---|
| | *Item* | *Benefit per year (RMB)* |
| Direct | Cost of O&M in wastewater treatment plant (residence rate 100%) | 68,024.320 (discharged flow: 80 l/person/day, community population: 2,912, average wastewater tariff: 0.8 RMB/$m^3$) [i] |
| | Income from reclaimed water (residence rate 100%) | 27,145.14 (flow: 82.634$m^3$/d, price of reclaimed water 1.0 RMB/$m^3$) [ii] |
| | Residual value | 181,143.147 (ratio of residual value: 4%) [iii] |
| External/ indirect | Decrease value of environment depravation from water pollution (residence rate 100%) | 400,493.18 (discharged flow: 80 l/person/day, community population: 2,912, value of environment deprivation 4.71 RMB/$m^3$ wastewater) [ix] |
| | **Cost of the project** | |
| | *Item* | *Cost per year (RMB)* |
| | Investment | 4,528,578.679 (calculation based on scale, treatment process, guidelines and other references. 40% of gross investment in first construction year, 60% in second year) [ii, iv, v, vi, xii] |
| | O&M | 134,948.30 (calculation based on scale, treatment process, guidelines and other references [ii, iv, v, vi, xii] |

i. China Reform and Development Committee, 2007
ii. Official reply on the price of reclaimed water in Baotou City, Inner Mongolia, China, September 2003 (in Chinese)
iii. Construction Ministry of China, 2006
iv. Shanghai Municipal Design Institute, 2000
v. Construction Ministry of China, 2001a
vi. Construction Ministry of China, 2001b
vii. Office of Underground Water Management in Dongsheng District, Erdos City, and Office of Water Saving in Dongsheng District, 2004
viii. Chen, 2003
ix. Chinese Environment Protection Agency and Chinese Statistics Bureau, 2004
x. Gao, 2002
xi. Zhou, 2001
xii. Construction Ministry of China, 2002a

**Table A.3** Economic criteria in EETP ecosan and conventional sanitation systems

| *Criterion* | *EETP ecosan system* | *Conventional sanitation system* |
|---|---|---|
| ENPV (social discount rate=8%) | 23,427,880.13 RMB | –1,449,793.74 RMB |

If the wastewater tariff were to be increased from 0.8 to 1.8 RMB/$m^3$ wastewater, the ENPV would be 325,468.25 RMB, which means the project would be accepted since the ENPV is greater than zero. After the wastewater tariff increase, the ENPV of the ecosan system becomes 95,546,913.49 RMB, which is still much more than the conventional sanitation system, thus the ecosan system is still accepted or feasible.

The social discount rate is not the same for all countries or organizations, for instance the social discount rate for the US is 1.6–3.2 per cent (for a time horizon of 3–30 years), while the social discount rate for the ADB (Asian Development Bank) region is 10–12 per cent. For environment protection projects in China, the guideline suggests that the social discount rate should be less than eight per cent (Construction Ministry of China, 2006). In this study, the ENPV of the ecosansystem is always greater than that of the conventional sanitation system, so the EETP ecosan system is acceptable from the country and societal considerations.

## Conclusions

Using a cost-benefit analysis (CBA) and a social discount rate of eight per cent, the ENPV of the ecosan system in the HZK community compared to the conventional sanitation system results in a ratio much greater than one, making the ecosan project feasible and accepted.

The ecosan system supplies a higher level of water savings, recycling of nutrients from human excreta, and reuse of wastewater. The total direct benefits from the ecosan system are 133,698.1 RMB/yr, which is 1.96 times more than the conventional sanitation system. External benefits that may be quantified are 14,178,159.91 RMB/yr, which is 35 times the conventional sanitation system.

Due to the fact that there are so few similar cases to learn from and that the technology and construction for urban multi-storey ecosan systems are still not standardized, the construction costs of the ecosan system were higher, i.e. 2.17 times that of the construction cost of the conventional sanitation system. It is believed that the construction cost for the ecosan system will decrease as the technology becomes more mature and with increased policy support.

The study showed that there are more benefits from externalities in the ecosan EETP project than in the conventional system. It is suggested that support mechanisms be developed including a water rights system, incentives for reduced wastewater discharge, and a rational wastewater tariff.

# Acknowledgements

A large number of individuals from China, Sweden, Germany, Japan, and the USA were involved in this project. An exhaustive list is not possible, but those that figured most in the project are listed here.

*Erdos Project Managers*: Zhang Dongsheng, Director of Erdos Planning Bureau; Han Yunxiang, Vice Chief of Dongsheng District Government; Sun Lixia, Director of Dongsheng Environment Protection Bureau (EPB).

*Erdos Project Administrative Assistant*: Li Jingrong, Vice Director of Dongsheng EPB.

*Erdos Project Administrative Office, Director*: Wang Zhigang, Dongsheng EPB.

*Erdos Project Administrative Office, Vice Director*: Shao Mingfeng, Dongsheng EPB.

*Erdos Project Administrative Office, secretarial assistant*: Kong Xiaofeng, Dongsheng EPB.

*Community Experts*: Ma Ling, Head of Tianjiao Street Office, Dongsheng District; Zheng Ping, Head of Tianjiao Community, Tianjiao Street Office, Dongsheng District; Wen Xiaohong, Head of Health Education Institute, Dongsheng Health Bureau; Sun Rongyong, Party Secretary of Tianjiao Community, Tianjiao Street Office.

*Eco-toilet and Eco-station Experts*: Zhang Yongfeng, PhD, Associate Professor, Chemical Engineering College of Inner Mongolia Polytechnic University; Chen Kebin, Managing Director, Meilong Industry.

*Greywater Experts*: Li Baolin, Engineer, Vice Director of Dongsheng EPB; Zhang Lijun, Engineer, Erdos Hongtu Construction, Survey & Design Corporation (Erdos Construction, Survey & Design Institute).

*Agriculture Reuse Expert*: Suo Quanyi, Professor, Inner Mongolia Agriculture University.

*Physical Infrastructure Experts*: Wen Zhi, Senior Engineer, Architect, Board-Chairman (Director) of ErdosHongtu Construction, Survey & Design Corporation; Wang Fenglian, Road Planner, Erdos Planning Bureau.

### Dongsheng District Personnel

*Project Office*: Director, Sun Lixia; Deputy Director, Li Rui; O&M and Accounting, Tian Dongming; Translator, Fu Rong; Secretary, Wang Qiang; Secretary, Zhang Mao; Social Worker, Ren Lingna; Technical Support, Mang Lai.

*Maintenance Team*: Chief, Lu Zhanrong; Workers: Liu Meifu, Chen Zhankui, Zhang Yijun, Liu Zirong, Xie Jushan, Wang Feiyun, Wang Lijun, Gao Meixiu, Zhang Xiunv, Qiao Fengfeng, Yan Min.

*SEI Personnel*: Project Supervisor, Arno Rosemarin; Assistant Supervisor, Guoyi Han; SEI Resident Project Manager, Xiao Jun; Senior Project Advisors: Uno Winblad, Zhu Qiang. Project Staff: Zhou Lele, Zhang Huiying, Feng Tongran, Hu Fengyi, Lin Bo, Zhang Weiwei.

*2007 International Sustainable Sanitation Conference in Dongsheng*: Ian Caldwell and Natasha Webster.

*External Research Experts/Consultants*: Zhang Zhiyang, Senior Engineer, TAES (greywater system design); Peter Ridderstolpe and Ebba af Petersens, Water Revival Systems (WRS), Uppsala (eco-toilet, greywater, and architectural aspects); Tang Runing, Professor, Inner Mongolia University of Polytechnology (ventilation study); Zhu Tianle, Professor, Beihang University and Beijing Aviation and Astronautic University (ventilation study and improvements); Zhou Lu, Professor Tsinghua Univ (cost-benefit analysis studies); Liu Zhong, Professor, Erdos Soil and Fertilizer Centre (agro reuse trials); Tang Yunping, Professor Tianjin Academy of Environmental Science (greywater treatment plant, design and training); Hidenori Harada, PhD, Kyoto University (ecosan expert, independent assessment); Wang Qingwang, Director, Lvhuanben Science and Technology Co. (composting plant design, construction, and training); Jan Mertens, Humboldt Univ Berlin (composting plant study); Mme Zhang Dongsheng, farmer in Erdos (reuse of compost in organic agriculture); Li Zifu (Professor) and Heinz-Peter Mang, Univ of Science and Technology in Beijing (project appraisal); Zhang Jian, PhD, EnviroSystems Engineering and Technology, Beijing (retrofitting of pipe systems); Wolfgang Berger, Berger-Biotechnik GmbH (ecosanitation systems specialist); Johannes Selke, Environmental Project Partners, Malaysia (pipe and plumbing specialist); Elisabeth Huba, World Toilet Organization (social systems expert); Kalle Rydberg and Wang Xin (toilet design and development); Scott Chen, Ecosan Consultant (Separett eco-toilets design and installation).

*Household Association*: Three representatives from the residents.

*Steering Committee of EETP*: Wang Bingjun, Vice Major of Erdos Municipality; Yang Hongyan, Party Secretary of the Dongsheng District; Zhao Wenliang, Governor of Dongsheng District; Sun Zhen, Chief of Environment Control Section, NDRC; Zhang Dongsheng, Director of Planning Bureau of Erdos Municipality; Yuan Zhigang, Deputy Party Secretary of Dongsheng District; Han Yunxiang, Vice Governor of Dongsheng District; Arno Rosemarin, SEI Project Supervisor; Uno Winblad, SEI Senior Advisor; Han Guoyi, SEI Associate Research Fellow; Zhu Qiang, SEI Senior Advisor; Xiao Jun, SEI Resident Consultant; Shi Zhongqin, Director of the EPB of Municipality; Sun Lixia, Director of the EPB of Dongsheng District; Wang Wanhou, Director of the Construction Bureau of Dongsheng District; Liu Yaochun, Director of the Land Bureau of Dongsheng District; GuoJiandong, Director of the Planning Bureau of Dongsheng; JiaYuping, Director of the Finance Bureau of Dongsheng District; Guo Lizhong, General Manager of Daxing Estate Development Co; Wen Zhi, Director of the Hongtu Design Institute.

# Notes

## Chapter 1

1. The Chinese Pinyin for the Ordos City is *Eerduosi*; derived from it, the short name Erdos was used for some time until the city decided to change it back to 'Ordos' in 2007, which is the name for the region commonly referred to in English literature. Given that in all the EETP project documents, the name Erdos was used, we continue to use it in this book.
2. China's 'Scientific Development Concept or Outlook' is a 'people-oriented' concept incorporating the goal of comprehensive, coordinated, and sustainable development, with the aim of achieving all-round economic, social and human progress (en.wikipedia.org).

## Chapter 3

1. NPV is the sum of the inflow and outflow of money (i.e. the net cost) and a discount rate based on the longevity of the investment.

## Annex 2

1. Contributors: Zhou Lu (zhou2001@263.net.cn) and Li Jian are with the Department of Environmental Science and Engineering, Tsinghua University, Beijing 100084, China. Zhu Qiang and Xiao Jun are with the China-Sweden Erdos Eco-Town Project, Dongsheng District, Erdos City, Inner-Mongolia 017000, China.

# References

(Project reports that are referred to as available from Stockholm Environment Institute can be accessed at www.ecosanres.org/erdos.htm)


Bai, Y.L. 2009. Personal communication. Secretary of Chinese Plant and Nutrition Institute; Researcher for Soil Aspects. Chinese Academy of Agricultural Sciences, Fertilizer Test Analysis Centre. 28 September.

Beijing Municipal Design Institute Design. 2000. *Manual for Water and Wastewater Engineering* (2nd edn) Vol.5. Wastewater Engineering. China Construction Industry Press, Beijing. (in Chinese)

Belli, P. *et al.*, 2001. *Economic Analysis of Investment Operations: Analytical Tools and Practical Applications.* World Bank, Washington, D.C.

Benidickson, J. 2007. *The Culture of Flushing: A Social and Legal History of Sewage.* UBC Press, Vancouver.

Berger, W. and Lorenz-Ladener, C. 2008. *Kompost-Toiletten. Sanitärsystem eohne Wasser (The Compost Toilet. Sanitation without Water).* Ökobuch Verlag.

Black, M. and Fawcett, B. 2008. *The Last Taboo: Opening the Door on the Global Sanitation Crisis.* Earthscan, UK and USA.

BORDA. 2009. *DEWATS.* Available from: <www.borda-net.org/modules/cjaycontent/index.php?id=29>

Capron, A., Dombrowicz, D. and Capron, M. 2004. 'Helminth infections and allergic diseases: From the paradigm to regulatory networks'. *Clinical Reviews in Allergy and Immunology.* 26(1): 25–35.

Chan, M. 1997. 'The global burden of intestinal nematode infections – fifty years on'. *Parasitology Today* 13: 438–43.

Chen, P. 2003. 'Analysis of reclaimed water application in China'. *Shanxi Architecture* 24(14): 80–81.

China Reform and Development Committee. 2007. *The General Work Plan for Energy Conservation and Pollutant Discharge Reduction.* (in Chinese)

Chinese Environment Protection Agency and Chinese Statistics Bureau. 2004. *China Green National Accounting Study Report 2004.* (in Chinese)

Chinese Environment Protection Agency. 2005. *China Environment Bulletin – 2006.*

Construction Ministry of China. 2001a. *Construction Standard of Urban Wastewater Engineering (revised edition).* China Planning Press, Beijing. (in Chinese)

Construction Ministry of China. 2001b. *Construction Standard of Sanitary Landfill for Urban Solid Waste.* China Planning Press, Beijing. (in Chinese)

Construction Ministry of China. 2002a. *Discharge Standards of Pollutants for Municipal Wastewater Treatment Plant.* (GB 18918-2002) (in Chinese)

Construction Ministry of China. 2002b. *Code for Design of Wastewater Reclamation and Reuse.* (GB50335-2002) (in Chinese)

Construction Ministry of China. 2002c. *Standard of Water Demand for Urban Resident*. (GB/T50331-2002) (in Chinese)

Construction Ministry of China. 2006. *Methods and Criterion (3rd edn)*. China Planning Press, Beijing. (in Chinese)

Dongsheng District Government. 2007. *Building a New Home – Sustainable Sanitation*. Video available from: <http://uk.youtube.com/watch?v=vvGbn0b1Tl4>.

EcoSanRes. 2004. 'Project Document: China–Sweden Erdos Eco-Town Project (EETP)'. EcoSanRes Program, Stockholm Environment Institute, Stockholm, Sweden.

Esrey, S.A., Gough, J., Rapaport, D. Sawyer, R., Simpson-Hébert, M., Vargas, J. and Winblad, U. (eds). 1998. *Ecological Sanitation*. Sida. Stockholm.

EWB. 2010. *Failure Report – Learning from Our Mistakes*. Engineers Without Borders. Canada. Available from: <http://legacy.ewb.ca/mainsite/pages/whoweare/accountable/FailureReport2011.pdf>

Flores, A. 2010.'Towards Sustainable Sanitation: Evaluating the Sustainability of Resource Oriented Sanitation'. Doctoral thesis, St. John's College, University of Cambridge.

Flores, A., Rosemarin, A. and Fenner, R. 2009. *Evaluating the Sustainability of an Innovative Dry Sanitation (Ecosan) System in China as Compared to a Conventional Waterborne Sanitation System*. In proceedings, WEFTEC, October, Florida.

Gao, Xiangzhao. 2002. *Manual of Fertilizer Usage*. China Agriculture Press, Beijing. (in Chinese)

George, R. 2008. *The Big Necessity: The Unmentionable World of Human Waste and Why It Matters*. Metropolitan Books, New York.

Government of Dongsheng District, Erdos Municipality. 2003. Introduction to Urban Development of the Dongsheng District. (in Chinese)

Haug, R.T. 1993. *The Practical Handbook of Compost Engineering*. Lewis Publishers, Boca Raton, FL.

Helmer, R. and Hespanhol, I. 1997. *Water Pollution Control*. WHO/UNEP.

Innovation Centre Denmark–Shanghai. 2009. *Wastewater Treatment in China*. Available from: <www.shanghai.um.dk/NR/rdonlyres/8483FA1C-DC53-4C7D-ADAB-E6148C25C99C/0/Industry_Analysis_Report11082009.pdf>

Jenkins, J. 2005. *The Humanure Handbook*. 3rd edn. Chelsea Green Publishing, Vermont.

Lingna, R. 2007. 'A Report on the Promotion of Ecosan System in Haozhaokui Daxing Community'. Presentation at the International Conference on Sustainable Sanitation: Eco-Cities and Villages, Dongsheng, Inner Mongolia, China, 26–31 August.

Liu, Z. 2007. 'Haozhaokui Community Ecosan System Research & Development Project Study on the Agricultural Application of Compost, Urine and Grey Water and Development & Demonstration'. Erdos Soil and Fertilizer Centre. Available from Stockholm Environment Institute.

Liu, Z. and Zhao, J. 2007. 'A preliminary study on the agricultural use of urban organic wastes and human excreta'. Erdos Soil and Fertilizer Centre and Inner Mongolia Academy of Agricultural Sciences. Presentation at the International Conference on Sustainable Sanitation: Eco-Cities and Villages, Dongsheng, Inner Mongolia, China, 26–31 August.

Lüthi, C., Panesar, A., Schütze, T., Norström, A., McConville, J., Parkinson, J., Saywell, D., and Ingle, R. 2010. *Sustainable Sanitation in Cities: A Framework for Action*. Papiroz Publishing House: Rijswiik, The Netherlands.

Ma, Y., Fan, S., Zhou, L., Dong, Z., Zhang, K. and Feng, J. 2007. 'The temporal change of driving factors during the course of land desertification in arid region of North China: the case of Minqin County'. *Environ Geol* 51: 999–1008.

Mara, D. 1998. 'Low-Cost Sewerage'. In: Simpson-Hébert, M. and Wood, S. (eds). *Sanitation Promotion, WSSCC Working Group on Promotion of Sanitation*. pp. 249–262. WHO, Geneva. WHO/EOS/98.5. Available from: <www.efm.leeds.ac.uk/CIVE/Sewerage/articles/WHO_EOS_98.5_pp249–262.pdf>

Mertens, J.H. 2009. 'Composting Project in the China Sweden Erdos Eco-Town'. Prepared as part of an internship with the Centre of Sustainable Environmental Sanitation at the University of Science and Technology Beijing (USTB).

Mertens, J. and Rosemarin, A. 2010. 'Producing organic fertiliser from urine-diverting dry toilets in Dongsheng, China'. *Urban Agriculture Magazine*. No. 23. April, p. 39.

Miguel, E. and Kremer, M. 2004. 'Worms: identifying impacts on education and health in the presence of treatment externalities'. *Econometrica* 72(1): 159–217.

Office of Underground Water Management in Dongsheng District, Erdos City and Office of Water Saving in Dongsheng District. 2004. *The Planning of Water Saving in Dongsheng District of Erdos City (2005 to 2010)*. (in Chinese)

Ordos On-line. 2010. *Profile of Ordos City*. Available from: <http://www.ordos.gov.cn/english/>

Palmqvist, H. and Jönsson, H. 2003. 'Urine, faeces, greywater, and biodegradable solid waste as potential fertilizers'. In proceedings, 1st IWA Conference on Sustainable Sanitation. 7–11 April, Lübeck.

Rosemarin, A. 2005. 'Sustainable sanitation and water in small urban centres'. *Water Science & Technology* 51(8): 109–118.

Rosemarin, A. 2007. 'The global sanitation crisis – why should 5000 dead children per day be a taboo subject?' *Loft Bookazine*, Stockholm, pp. 278–285.

Rosemarin, A. 2009. 'Dry and WET! Sanitation in Multi-Storey Apartment Buildings: The Case of Dongsheng, Erdos, Inner Mongolia, China'. Presented at the 2009 Dry Toilet Conference, 13–15 August, Tampere, Finland.

Rosemarin, A., Ekane, N., Caldwell, I., Kvarnström, E., McConville, J., Ruben, C. and Fogde, M. 2008. *Pathways for Sustainable Sanitation: Achieving the Millennium Development Goals*. IWA, London.

Rosemarin, A., de Bruijne, G. and Caldwell, I. 2009. 'Peak phosphorus: the next inconvenient truth'. *The Broker Issue* 15: 6–9.

Rosemarin, A., Cordell, D., Dagerskog, L., Smit, A.L. and Schröder, J.J. 2010. *Maximising Recycling Opportunities for Phosphate and Other Nutrients*. International Fertiliser Society, Cambridge, December.

Scott, C.A., Faruqui, N.I. and Raschid-Sally, L. 2004. *Wastewater Use in Irrigated Agriculture: Coordinating the Livelihood and Environmental Realities*. CABI/IWMI/IDRC. Available from: <www.idrc.ca/en/ev-31595-201-1-DO_TOPIC.html>

Selke, J. 2008. Report: 'Working Visit to China Sweden Erdos Eco – City Town Project'. Prepared for: EcoSanRes, Stockholm Environment Institute Stockholm, Sweden.

Shalizi, Z. 2006. 'Addressing China's growing water shortages and associated social and environmental consequences'. World Bank Policy Research Working Paper 3895. Washington, D.C.: The World Bank.

Shanghai Municipal Design Institute. 2000. 'Design manual for water and wastewater engineering' (2nd edn) Vol.10. *Engineering Economics*, China Construction Industry Press, Beijing. (in Chinese)

Stenström, T.A., Seidu, R., Ekane, N. and Zurbrügg, C. 2011. 'Microbial Exposure and Health Assessments in Sanitation Technologies and Systems'. *EcoSanRes Series* 2011-1. Stockholm Environment Institute. Available from: <www.ecosanres.org/pdf_files/Microbial_Exposure_&_Health_Assessments_in_Sanitation_Technologies_&_Systems.pdf>

SuSanA (Sustainable Sanitation Alliance). 2008. 'Towards more sustainable sanitation solutions', Version 1.2. Available from: <http://susana.org/lang-en/intro/156-intro/267-vision-document> [accessed 28 November 2010].

Tilley, E., Lüthi, C., Morel, A., Zurbrügg, C. and Schertenleib, R. 2008. *Compendium of Sanitation Systems and Technologies*. Swiss Federal Institute of Aquatic Science and Technology (EAWAG). Switzerland.

Ujang, Z. and Henze, M. (eds). 2006. *Municipal Wastewater Management in Developing Countries*. Principles and Engineering, IWA, London.

UNFPA. 2007. *State of the World Population: Unleashing the Potential of Urban Growth*. United Nations Population Fund, New York.

UN Habitat. 2008. *State of the World's Cities 2008/2009*. Earthscan, London.

UNESCO. 2006. *Water, a Shared Responsibility*. Berghahn Books, New York.

Vinnerås, B., Palmquist, H., Balmer, P. and Jönsson, H. 2006. 'The characteristics of household wastewater and biodegradable solid waste – A proposal for new Swedish design values'. *Urban Water* 3(1): 3–11.

World Health Organization (WHO). 2006. *WHO guidelines for the safe use of wastewater, excreta and greywater, Volume IV Excreta and greywater use in agriculture*. WHO Press, Geneva, Switzerland.

WHO & UNICEF. 2008. *Progress on drinking water and sanitation. Special focus on sanitation*. WHO Press, Geneva, Switzerland.

WHO & UNICEF. 2010. *Progress on Sanitation and Drinking-Water*, 2010 Update. WHO, Geneva, Switzerland.

Want China Times, 2011. 'Housing bubble in Inner Mongolia's Ordos bursts'. Available from: <www.wantchinatimes.com/news-subclass-cnt.aspx?id=20110711000005&cid=1102>

Williams, P.T. 2005. *Waste Treatment and Disposal*. Wiley and Sons, USA.

Williams, A.P., Avery, L.M., Killham, K., and Jones, D.L. 2008. 'Moisture, sawdust, and bleach regulate the persistence of Escherichia coli O157:H7 on floor surfaces in butcher shops'. *Food Control*, 19(2008), 1119–1125.

Winblad, U. and Simpson-Hébert, M. (eds). 2004. *Ecological Sanitation*, revised. Stockholm Environment Institute, Stockholm.

Woodworth, M.D. 2011. 'Frontier boomtown urbanism in Ordos, Inner Mongolia Autonomous Region'. In: *Cross-Currents: East Asian History and Culture Review*. E-Journal 1(1) (December 2011). Available from:

<http://cross-currents.berkeley.edu/sites/default/files/e-journal/articles/woodworth_0.pdf>

World Bank. 2005. 'Erdos Urban Region Development Strategy. A Report to the Municipal People's Government of Erdos. China: City-Region Development Strategies 2 Project'. Prepared by Chreod Ltd, Ottawa.

World Bank. 2007. *Stepping Up: Improving the Performance of China's Urban Water Utilities*. World Bank, Washington D.C.

World Population Prospects. 2006. Available from: <www.un.org/esa/population/publications/wpp2006/wpp2006.htm>

Zhou, L. 2001. *Engineering economic and cost management in environment engineering*, Chemical Industry Press, Beijing. (in Chinese)

Zhou, L., Li, J., Yu, C., and Wang, Y. 2007. 'Erdos Eco-Town Project of Inner Mongolia: Economic Evaluation of the Ecosan System'. Available from EcoSanRes, Stockholm Environment Institute, Stockholm, Sweden.

Zhu, Q. 2008. 'Report on Technical Summary of the China–Sweden Erdos Eco-Town Project – From February 2003 to July 2007'. Available from EcoSanRes, Stockholm Environment Institute, Stockholm, Sweden.

Zhu, T. 2007. 'A Study on Reconstruction for Ventilation System of Dry-toilet at Haozhaokui Community of Erdos City'. Beihang University. Available from Stockholm Environment Institute.

www.ingramcontent.com/pod-product-compliance
Ingram Content Group UK Ltd.
Pitfield, Milton Keynes, MK11 3LW, UK
UKHW061829100926
8556IPUK00010B/925
* 9 7 8 1 8 5 3 3 9 7 6 7 7 *